Advanced Topics in Artery Bypass

Advanced Topics in Artery Bypass

Edited by **Jessica Clan**

FOSTER
ACADEMICS

New Jersey

Published by Foster Academics,
61 Van Reypen Street,
Jersey City, NJ 07306, USA
www.fosteracademics.com

Advanced Topics in Artery Bypass
Edited by Jessica Clan

International Standard Book Number: 978-1-63242-029-9 (Hardback)

Printed in the United States of America.

Contents

Permissions

List of Contributors

Preface

This book has been an outcome of determined endeavour from a group of educationists in the field. The primary objective was to involve a broad spectrum of professionals from diverse cultural background involved in the field for developing new researches. The book not only targets students but also scholars pursuing higher research for further enhancement of the theoretical and practical applications of the subject.

This book examines diagnostic and therapeutic modalities in the management of coronary artery disease by percutaneous coronary intervention with stenting and in the interventional management of other atherosclerotic vascular disease, which have led to a decline in cardiovascular mortality and morbidity. Also, the book discusses cardiac surgical topics. This book, written by experts in their fields, offers a wonderful update on the developments which every physician treating their patients with atherosclerotic vascular disease should be acquainted with.

It was an honour to edit such a profound book and also a challenging task to compile and examine all the relevant data for accuracy and originality. I wish to acknowledge the efforts of the contributors for submitting such brilliant and diverse chapters in the field and for endlessly working for the completion of the book. Last, but not the least; I thank my family for being a constant source of support in all my research endeavours.

Editor

Percutaneous Coronary Intervention

Generating Graphical Reports on Cardiac Catheterization

Yuki Igarashi, Takeo Igarashi, Ryo Haraguchi and
Kazuo Nakazawa

Additional information is available at the end of the chapter

1. Introduction

Electronic medical recording systems [1-4] have become widespread due to the improvement in hardware performance and user interfaces. Some recent systems are designed to support doctor–patient communication using a tablet PC [5-6]. However, usability is still an issue and medical professionals need more such user-friendly interfaces. To make these systems accessible to inexperienced users and to reduce the overhead of data entry, we have been developing various pen-based electronic medical recording systems [7-8]. Pen-based computing is an active research area for both user interfaces and computer graphics. Our work is based on recent advances in this area, especially the freeform user interfaces proposed by Igarashi [9]. Using this approach, the user draws freehand lines on the screen assisted by the system, and the result is directly stored as a vector image. Our systems feature special purpose functions for pen input including three-dimensional (3D) sketching, user-identification, and handwritten character recognition and search [8]. They are designed to help medical professionals to think more freely when working on difficult problems without being constrained by cumbersome interfaces.

One problem with these freeform pen-based systems, however, is that their output does not easily fit into a structure that lends itself to further machine processing or interface with other more traditional recording systems. Our goal in the project was to bridge this gap between freeform diagramming and more structured recording.

One strength of pen-based systems is that they make it easy to draw and add diagrams to medical records. This is particularly useful in ophthalmology, otolaryngology, and dentistry in which diagrams play an important role in medical records. Indeed, the frequent use of diagrams makes it difficult to use traditional GUI-based medical recording systems in these areas [10]. Cardiac catheterization is one of these areas in which the diagram is an indispensable tool for medical recording. Existing electronic medical recording systems rely on structured templates, but it is difficult to create an appropriate report of findings or treatment plan using these predefined templates. Most existing diagram editors are implemented as bitmap paint tools, not vector graphics. This makes it difficult to edit the geometry afterward and requires that a large amount of data be transmitted and stored

We therefore developed a pen-based interface for graphical reporting of findings in cardiac catheterization (Figure 1) [11]. Figure 2 shows an illustration of the human heart. The target of our system is the coronary arteries. Figure 3 shows a screenshot of our system. The user can freely "sketch" coronary arteries and stenoses on the screen using a pen on a template of coronary features. The location and degree of each stenosis, and various treatments such as bypass and stents, are visually represented. We developed an algorithm that can extract semantic information from the graphical representation and store it in XML format. The system can also generate a table in the format specified in the AHA (American Heart Association) committee report [12]. This system is useful not only as a tool for efficiently generating reports of findings but also as an effective explanation tool for patients.

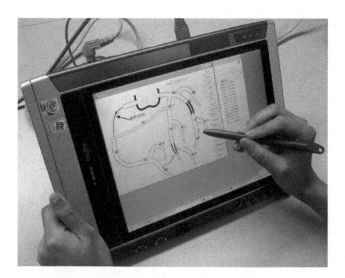

Figure 1. A screenshot of our system in use.

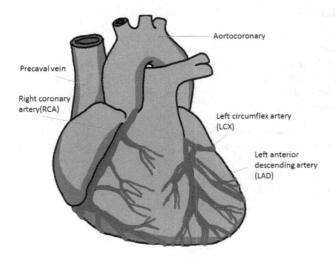

Figure 2. An illustration of the human heart. The target of our system is the coronary arteries (the red vessels shown in this figure).

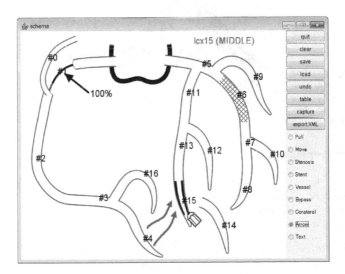

Figure 3. Recording an example of cardiac catheterization.

2. User Interface

The user can draw on the diagram template using a pen as if drawing on real paper. Our system shows the name of each coronary artery and segment (e.g., proximal, middle, or distal) at the upper right of the screen when the cursor is over any vessel. We use the naming scheme defined in the AHA committee report. The system can show border lines of coronary artery segments if required.

Our system is a Windows application that provides a familiar interface to permit new users to work with it without extensive training. For example, the system displays a pop-up menu when the user clicks on a window while pressing the barrel button on the pen (Figure 4). This section describes the user interaction steps one by one. The next section describes our algorithm.

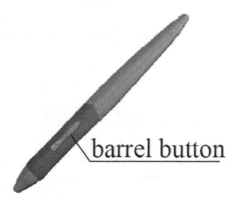

Figure 4. Barrel button on pen.

2.1. Insertion / editing of a vessel

Upon start-up, our system displays a default cardiac catheterization coronary schema. The user can then draw a finding report or a treatment plan on the schema. The system provides several functions for editing the geometry on screen, including adding, deleting, and deforming arteries.

The user can draw a new coronary artery with the pen after choosing the "draw coronary artery" mode from the tool palette on the right (Figure 5 (a)). The system automatically creates an appropriate junction where the new artery is connected to another, and tapers the free end. The user can delete a vessel by clicking on it while holding the barrel button down and choosing "delete" from a pop-up menu. The system automatically updates the display on the screen. The user can move an artery by dragging it with the pen after choosing the "move coronary artery" mode from the tool palette (Figure 5 (b)). The user can deform an artery by dragging it with the pen (Figure 5 (c)) after choosing the "pull coronary artery" mode from the tool palette. We use a pulling interface for a curve that was introduced in [13]. It deforms a curve while preserving the local geometry. The user can also set the line width to small, normal, or large, using a pop-up panel (Figure 6). This system also supports the `absent' display, as shown in Figure 7.

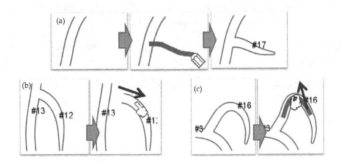

Figure 5. Editing operations on a coronary artery. (a) Draw a new coronary artery; (b) Move a coronary artery; (c) Pull a coronary artery

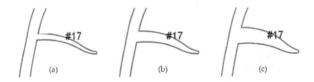

Figure 6. The user can set the line width to small, normal, or large, using a pop-up panel. (a) Small; (b) Normal; (c) Large

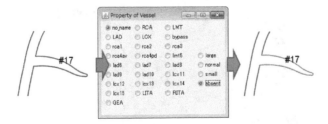

Figure 7. The system also supports the `absent' display

2.2. Recording of stenoses

Once the user has sketched the geometry of the coronary arteries, he or she can record stenoses. To do this, the user chooses the "draw stenosis" mode from the tool palette and draws the stenosis on the target artery with the pen (Figure 8 (a)). When the user completes drawing and lifts the pen from the screen, the system displays a dialog box to specify the type and severity of the stenosis (Figure 8 (b)). If the user wants to change the properties of an existing stenosis, he or she can open the properties window by clicking on the affected artery while holding the barrel button down. The display of each stenosis on the screen includes the severity specified by the user (Figure 8 (c)).

The user can also move an existing stenosis by dragging it along the coronary artery (Figure 9). The stenosis snaps to the border of the appropriate section of the artery as it moves.

If the severity of a stenosis is set to 100%, the portion of the artery beyond the stenosis is shown as a thin line (Figure 10 (a)) representing a complete blockage where no blood flows. The system automatically analyzes the tree structure of arteries and closes any downstream vessels as well.

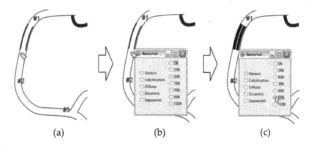

(a)   (b)   (c)

Figure 8. Recording a stenosis. When the user draws a stenosis (a), the system displays a dialog box to specify the type and severity of the stenosis (b, c).

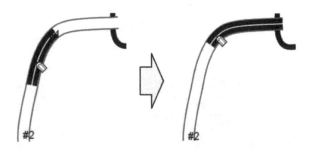

Figure 9. The user can move an existing stenosis by dragging it along the coronary artery.

2.3. Bypasses and collateral

The user can add a bypass to the schema by drawing a line connecting coronary arteries. If the bypass connects an open artery to a closed one, the system automatically opens the blockage to indicate that blood flow has been restored (Figure 10 (b)). The user can place a stenosis on a bypass just like on a coronary artery and can also delete, move, and pull a bypass.

The user can draw a collateral (new blood vessels that reroute blood flow around a stenosis) by drawing a line between coronary arteries. This appears as an arrow in the schema (Figure 11). Our current implementation does not modify the blood flow automatically in response to a new collateral.

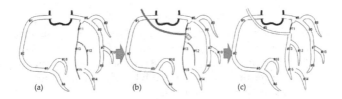

(a)   (b)   (c)

Figure 10. Drawing a bypass. If the bypass connects an open coronary artery to a closed one (a), the system automatically opens the closed coronary artery to indicate that blood flow has resumed (b, c).

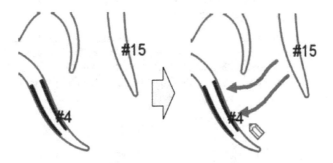

Figure 11. Example of recording a collateral.

2.4. Stent

The user can place a stent in a coronary artery (Figure 12). Recording of stents is very important for documenting the treatment of the stenosis. The procedure for editing a stent is identical to that for editing a stenosis. The user creates and moves a stent by dragging it along a coronary artery and deletes it using a pop-up menu. The stent also snaps to the borders of the artery segments.

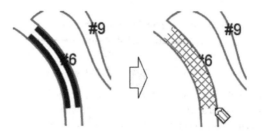

Figure 12. Example of placing a stent.

2.5. Other Functions

The user can annotate the schema as a record of miscellaneous medical diagnosis and treat-ment. Our current implementation supports text and arrow marks in annotations (Figure 13). Unconstrained annotation encourages the user to think freely, similar to handwriting notes on traditional paper medical records. It is also helpful to remind the user of miscella-neous details associated with specific treatments.

The system can save an edited coronary schema, and then load it again for review or further editing. The schema is stored as vector graphics to reduce file size and facilitate editing. The system can export a schema in PNG image format for import into another system.

The user can create a new schema starting from a default coronary schema template and can also specify any schema to be the default template.

When the user places the mouse cursor on a vessel, the system displays the name of the ves-sel at the top right corner of the screen, as shown in Figure 14. The system displays not only the name of the vessel, but also its position ('PROXIMAL', 'MIDDLE' or 'DISTAL') in each blood vessel. Moreover, segment border lines are displayed when the user enables this fea-ture in the pop-up menu shown in Figure 15.

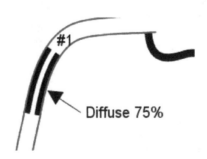

Figure 13. Example of recording text and arrow marks as an annotation.

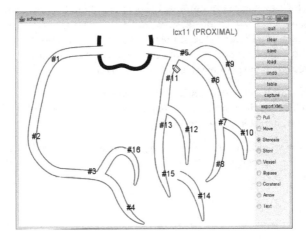

Figure 14. The system displays the name of the vessel at the top right of the screen when the user places the mouse cursor over it.

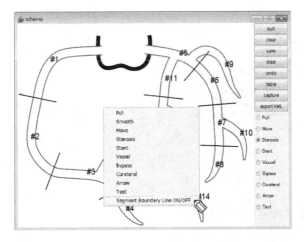

Figure 15. The system displays segment border lines when the user enables this feature in the pop-up menu.

3. Dataset structure and cooperation with other systems

Many doctors use coronary angiography (CAG) to represent coronary stenosis pathology. CAG compactly shows the location and severity of stenoses. Our system supports the conversion of the graphical record to a CAG-compliant table dataset. The table is represented in the format specified in the AHA committee report and stored as an XML file. Figure 16 shows the relationship between our system and CAG. The top screen in Figure 16 (a) presents an example of recording stenoses using our system; the middle screen of Figure 16 (a) shows the CAG dataset it produces. Any other system that supports this format can use the data file as shown in the bottom screen of Figure 16 (a).

The user can also edit the exported CAG table. When this happens, our system automatically updates the corresponding stenosis on the coronary diagram including the information on the severity and character of the stenosis (Figure 16 (b)).

When a stenosis is straddling two or more segments, it is considered to belong to two or more segments. The stenosis drawn on LAD7 and LAD8 amid the strangulation shown in Figure 17 is an example.

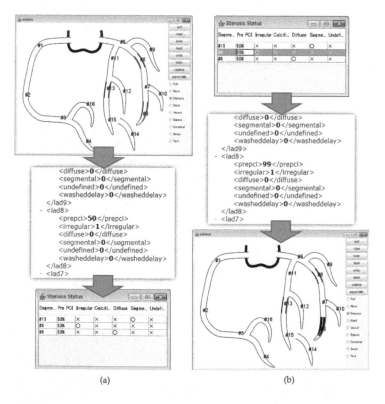

(a)   (b)

Figure 16. Example of the automatic relationship between the coronary diagram and the CAG table. (a) The system automatically generates a CAG table from a graphical coronary schema by checking the existence of a stenosis in each segment of the coronary arteries, and stores the results in XML format. (b) The system can automatically update the stenoses on the coronary schema from the corresponding CAG table.

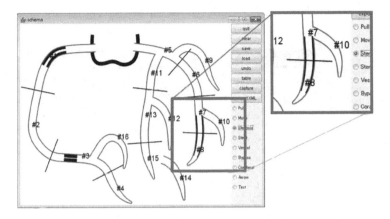

Figure 17. Example of a stenosis over two divisions.

4. Implementation

We designed our system as a platform-independent Java™ program using the Java2D™ graphics application programming interface. This section describes the implementation details of the current prototype.

4.1. On-screen displays

The system displays coronary arteries as two parallel lines and handles the branches appropriately (Figure 18 (a)). A vessel is a polyline composed of small line segments. The system first draws a wide red line and then a narrow white line inside (Figure 18 (b1), (b2)). The width of these lines decreases toward the non-connected end of a vessel to represent the taper (Figure 18 (c1), (c2)).

A stenosis is displayed in a similar manner. The system first draws a wide black line inside the vessel and then a narrow white line inside that. A stent is rendered by drawing a hatching pattern after setting a stencil inside the stent area.

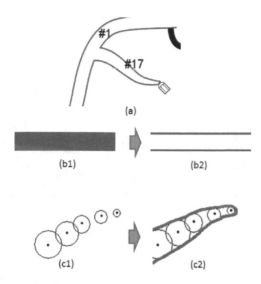

Figure 18. Vessel representation. The system displays coronary arteries as two parallel lines and handles the branches appropriately (a). The system first draws a wide red line (b1), and then a narrow white line inside (b2). The width of these lines decreases toward the non-connected end of a vessel to represent the taper (c1, c2).

4.2. Geometry editing

The pulling interface deforms the curve while maintaining its local details (Figure 5 (c)) [13]. The system first generates triangles by connecting sets of three neighboring points on a polyline. As the user pulls a point along the curve, the system determines the location of free vertices so as to minimize the distortion of the triangles. We also used the peeling interface introduced in [13] to adjust the size of the region to be deformed, so that a larger area is deformed as the user pulls more. As the user pulls the curve further away, the influence region grows (Figure 19, left to right).

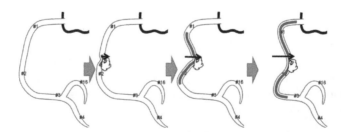

Figure 19. We use the pulling and peeling interface introduced in [13]. As the user pulls the curve further away, the influence region grows (left to right).

4.3. Generation of the CAG table

The CAG table stores the following information for each segment of a coronary artery: the presence or absence of a stenosis, the severity of the stenosis, and the type of stenosis (Figure 16 (a), bottom). The system automatically generates a CAG table from a graphical coronary schema by checking for the existence of a stenosis in each segment. It stores the result in XML format (Figure 16 (a), middle and bottom).

When the user edits the CAG table, the system first finds the corresponding stenosis in the XML file (Figure 16 (b), top and middle). It then obtains the information for that stenosis and changes it on the coronary schema. In this way, the system automatically updates the stenoses on the coronary schema from the corresponding CAG table (Figure 16 (b), bottom).

5. Case report using our system

We illustrate the effectiveness of our system, utilizing two cases of coronary artery bypass surgery as examples. These examples were only described (not illustrated) in the original papers.

The first example is Case 1 of [14]. The paper describes it as follows:

`A man, 45 years of age, had suffered attacks of angina pectoris during many years. He had had infarction of the myocardium. During the operation it was noted that the left coronary artery and the initial portions of its main branches were calcified. We also noted density of the right coronary artery. Anastomosis was applied between the inner thoracic artery and the circumflex branch of the left coronary artery.'

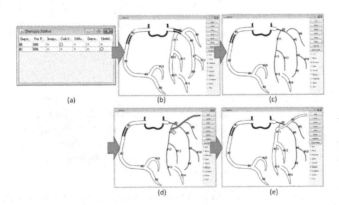

Figure 20. Case 1 of the report [14] using our system.

Figure 20 shows how to illustrate this process using our system. First, the user inputs a CAG table, as shown in Figure 20 (a). With our system, the user can set the type of the corresponding stenosis, as shown in the CAG table. The system then automatically generates a graphical coronary schema, as shown in Figure 20 (b). Figure 20 (c) shows the result of setting the severity of a stenosis of the left coronary artery to 100%.

The bypass connects an open vessel to the closed coronary artery, and the system automatically opens the closed coronary artery to indicate that blood flow is recovered, as shown in Figure 20 (d, e).

The second example is Case 3 of the report [14]. The paper describes it as follows:

`A male patient (40 years of age), had suffered from generalized atherosclerosis. (…) During the operation calcification and complete occlusion of the initial portion of both branches of the left coronary artery were found. An end-to-end anastomosis between the inner thoracic and interventricular arteries was made.'

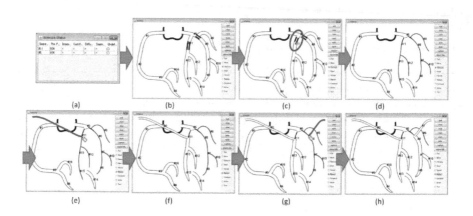

Figure 21. Case 3 of the report [14] using our system.

Figure 21 shows how to illustrate this process using our system. First, the user inputs a CAG table, as shown in Figure 21 (a). The system then automatically generates a graphical coronary schema, as shown in Figure 21 (b). By default, the system automatically generates the stenosis in the middle portion of the corresponding vessel, as shown in Figure 21 (b). The user can move the stenosis to the initial portion, as shown in Figure 21 (c). Figure 21 (d) shows the result of setting the severity of the stenosis to 100%.

The bypass connects an open vessel to the closed coronary artery, and the system automatically opens the closed coronary artery to indicate that blood flow is recovered, as shown in Figure 21 (e, f) and (g, h).

6. Discussion

Our current implementation is a research prototype and is not yet being used in clinical practice. However, we have already demonstrated it to medical professionals and confirmed the following benefits:

1. The user can easily modify the geometry of coronary arteries for individual patients.

2. The system can store the data compactly using vectors instead of bitmaps, which significantly improves the network response when storing information on a remote server.

3. The system can export the CAG table based on the AHA committee report in XML format. Therefore, the system can easily exchange data with other existing systems.

4. The user can edit a coronary schema while viewing a reference image on the same display.

5. The user can draw diagrams and text freely in our system, which allows the recording of new anomalies that have never been previously observed.

In addition, we received the following comment from another heart surgeon: `This is a user-friendly system. It is particularly effective for inexperienced doctors. Diagnosis is performed by a heart physician. But, I think that it is useful also for a young surgeon's training.'

The correspondence between a diagnosis and a dissection, as well as comparison between the diagnosis and a CT scan image, are important to a surgeonpreparing for an operation. However, even though there is an AHA standard that defines how to verbalize diagnosis results, there is significant variation in the way surgeons describe diagnosis results, even among experts. Accordingly, one specialist commented that it is useful to have a link between CT scan images of the circumflex branches to the corresponding locations in the schema. The specialist also commented that two-dimensional (2D) representation is sufficient if the purpose of the target system is diagnosis, but 3D representation is desirable for training purposes.

An issue with the current implementation is that it is limited by the AHA standards. The manner of recording schemas for cardiac catheterization varies widely among users and facilities. As the AHA committee report was designed more than 30 years ago, it cannot handle many cases well. Therefore, a more powerful and flexible representation is needed.

7. Conclusion and future work

We developed an effective interface for reporting graphical findings in cardiac catheterization using hand-drawn diagrams. The user can easily record the position and degree of a stenosis on a coronary schema template, and can also record treatments such as bypasses and stents. Once a bypass is added, the system automatically displays the resumption of blood flow. This type of automatic adaptation is not possible with paper-based medical records. Our system can store the data as a CAG table in an XML file in the AHA format for exchanging data with other existing systems. Our system makes it easier to handle graphical schemas in medical recording systems, encouraging the spread of medical recording systems in general.

Our system operates independently and does not require any other special infrastructure. Therefore, it can be easily introduced at low cost. We hope to put our system into actual clinical practice to make improvements based on feedback from actual users. We also plan to experiment with 3D schemas because 3D images are becoming increasingly widespread. We are also currently working with methods pertaining to 3D images. For example, Nakao et al. proposed a 3D cardiovascular modeling system based on neonatal echocardiographic images [15]. Using this system, medical doctors can interactively construct patient-specific cardiovascular models, and share the complex topology and shape information. Bo et al. introduced a lightweight sketching system that enables interactive illustration of complex fluid systems [16]. Users can sketch on a 2.5D canvas to design the shapes and connections of a fluid circuit. Ijiri et al. developed an efficient and robust framework for simulating the cardiac beating motion [17]. The global cardiac motion is generated by the accumulation of local myocardial fiber contractions. They compute such local-to-global deformations using a kinematic approach, dividing a heart mesh model into overlapping local regions, contracting them independently according to fiber orientation, and computing a global shape that fits the contracted shapes of all local regions as well as possible.

The interactive graphical schemas introduced in this paper should be useful in not only cardiac catheterization but also other areas that use schemas, for example, ophthalmology, otolaryngology, and dentistry. Such interactive schemas are useful not only for efficiently generating finding reports but also as an effective explanation tool for patients.

Author details

Yuki Igarashi[1], Takeo Igarashi[2], Ryo Haraguchi[3] and Kazuo Nakazawa[3]

1 University of Tsukuba, Japan

2 The University of Tokyo, Japan

3 National Cerebral and Cardiovascular Center Reserch Institute, Japan

References

[1] Takashi Matsumura. Electronic Medical Record and Hospital Information System . Comprehensive Management of Patient Information--. Japan Journal of Medical Informatics, 21(3), 2001, 211-222 (in Japanese).

[2] Yasushi Matsumura. Current Status of Electronic Medical Record and its Tasks. The Medical Frontline, 2003; 58(8): 46-51 (in Japanese).

[3] Dean F. Sitting, Gilad J. Kuperman, Julie Fiskio. Evaluating Physician Satisfaction Regarding User Interactions with an Electronic Medical Record System. Proceedings of AMIA Annual Symposium 99, 1999, 400-404.

[4] Mark Ginsburg. Pediatric Electronic Health Record Interface Design: The PedOne System. Proceedings of the 40th Hawaii International Conference on System Sciences, 2007, 139.

[5] Erik K. Fromme, Tawni Kenworthy-Heinige and Michelle Hribar. Developing an easy-to-use tablet computer application for assessing patient-reported outcomes in patients with cancer. Supportive Care in Cancer, Volume 19, Number 6 (2011), 815-822.

[6] Ole Andreas Alsos, Anita Das, Dag Svanæs. Mobile health IT: The effect of user inter face and form factor on doctor–patient communication. International Journal of Medical Informatics, 81(1), 12-28, 2012.

[7] Kazuo Nakazawa, Takeo Igarashi. A Comprehensive Computer Interface for the Spreading of Electronic Medical Recording Systems Supporting Hand-writing Inputs by Pen Device. New Medicine in Japan, 2003; 345: 74-77 (in Japanese).

[8] Kazuo Nakazawa, Ryo Haraguchi, Takenori Yao, Satoru Nagata, Yoshihisa Sugimoto, Takashi Ashihara, Masahiro Takada, Hirokazu Namikawa, Yasushi Okada, Kohei Yoshimoto, Naomi Furuya, Shuji Senda, Yoshiyuki Ucmatsu, Takeo Igarashi. Pen-based Interface for Electronic Medical Record System with Advanced Recognition and Search Engine for the Hand-written Characters. Japan Journal of Medical Informatics, 2005; 25(2), 81-86 (in Japanese).

[9] Takeo Igarashi, "Freeform User Interfaces for Graphical Computing", Proceedings of 3rd International Symposium on Smart Graphics, Lecture Notes in Computer Science, Springer, 39-48, 2003.

[10] Sakabe Nagamasa, Arai Kazuo, Abe Kazuya, Inoue Hideo, Sakai Shunichi, Watanabe Yukio. A Survey of demerits of Electronic Medical Record in the Ear-Nose and Throat Department. Japan Journal of Medical Informatics, 2001; 21(1): 131-136 (in Japanese).

[11] Yuki Mori, Takeo Igarashi, Ryo Haraguchi, and Kazuo Nakazawa. A Pen-based Interface for Generating Graphical Reports of Findings in Cardiac Catheterization. Methods of Information in Medicine, 2007;46(6) pp.694-699.

[12] Austen G. W, Eswards J, Frye R. L., et al. "A Reporting System on Patients Evaluated for Coronary Artery Disease", Circulation, 1975; 51(4 Suppl.): 5-40.

[13] Igarashi T, Moscovich T, Hughes J F. As-Rigid-As-Possible Shape Manipulation. ACM Transactions on Computer Graphics 2005; 24(3): 1134-1141

[14] Kolessov, V. I. Mammary artery-coronary artery anastomosis as method of treatment for angina pectoris. The Journal of Thoracic and Cardiovascular Surgery. 1967; 54(4): 535-544.

[15] Megumi Nakao, Kazuma Maeda, Ryo Haraguchi, Ken-ichi Kurosaki, Koji Kagisaki, Isao Shiraishi, Kazuo Nakazawa, Kotaro Minato. "Cardiovascular Modeling of Congenital Heart Disease Based on Neonatal Echocardiographic Images", IEEE Transactions on Information Technology in BioMedicine, 16(1), 70-79, 2012.

[16] Bo Zhu, Michiaki Iwata, Ryo Haraguchi, Takashi Ashihara, Nobuyuki Umetani, Takeo Igarashi, Kazuo Nakazawa. Sketch-based Dynamic Illustration of Fluid Systems. ACM Transactions on Graphics (Proceedings of SIGGRAPH Asia 2011), 30(6), Article No. 134, 2011.

[17] Ijiri T, Ashihara T, Umetani N, Igarashi T, Haraguchi R, et al. (2012) A Kinematic Approach for Efficient and Robust Simulation of the Cardiac Beating Motion. PLoS ONE 7(5): e36706.

Chapter 2

Multivessel Disease in the Modern Era of Percutaneous Coronary Intervention

Michael Tsang and JD Schwalm

Additional information is available at the end of the chapter

1. Introduction

The rapid evolution of medical therapy, percutaneous coronary interventional techniques and cardiac surgery along with the changing patient profile over the last few decades has required the clinician to make increasingly complex decisions. This has led to significant variations in practices that may be discordant with evidence based clinical practice guidelines. Such variations have an unclear clinical impact. There is hope that with growing efforts to apply multidisciplinary care to the management of complex coronary artery disease (CAD),that we will arrive at more consistent and balanced decisions.

In this chapter, we will explore (1) The history of angiography and angioplasty, (2) the current clinical dilemma (3) the evidence supporting the use of cardiac surgery to improve survival above medical therapy alone, (4) the role of percutaneous approach versus surgery in different populations, (5) the impact of changing technologies/techniques in revascularization, (6) the current discordance between guidelines and clinical practice, and (7) the potential role of a multidisciplinary Heart Team to create a more unified, balanced approach to the treatment of complex CAD.

2. The origins of the age of percutaneous revascularization

2.1. Cardiac catheterization

One of the earliest descriptions of cardiac catheterizations was done by Steven Hales, an English chemist, botanist and animal physiologist who cannulated the carotid artery and the jugular vein to access the left and right-sided chambers of the heart respectively in the 17th century [1]. It was through some of this initial work, that he was able to make the first measurements of blood pressure, describe systole and diastole, characterize the volumes of the heart through wax cast work and correctly describe the function of the aortic and mitral valve [1]. Interestingly, the first human cardiac catheterization was by a Urologist by the name of Werner Forssmann [2]. He performed right heart catheterization on himself in 1929 by advancing a cannula through the left antecubital vein via cut-down access into the right atrium [2].

2.2. Selective coronary angiography and angioplasty

The credit of the first true selective coronary angiogram and much of the initial correlations between angina pectoris and coronary anatomy has to be granted to Mason Sones, a Pediatric Cardiologist, who at the time of discovery was working out of the Cleveland clinic [3-5]. In 1958, whilst performing non-selective aortogram on a patient, Sones inadvertently engaged the right coronary artery [2].

The original technique of angioplasty was born out earlier work by a Vascular Radiologist by the name of Charles Theodore Dotter [6]. Andreas Gruentzig, now known as the father of modern day coronary angioplasty, learned the Dotter technique from a German Radiologist Eberard Zeitler while doing a clinical fellowship in the Radiology Department of Aggertalclinic in Engelskirchen, Germany [6]. He had adopted the Dotter concept of using the balloon approach for angioplasty [6]. After experimenting with a number of materials performed the first procedure in 1977 in a man with stenosis of his left anterior descending artery (LAD) using a polyvinyl chloride balloon mounted onto the Dotter catheter [6].

3. The current dilemma

The treatment of coronary artery disease can be simplified into three major therapeutic approaches: medical therapy alone, percutaneous coronary intervention (PCI), and coronary artery bypass grafting (CABG). However, deciding on which approach is optimal for the individual patient is sometimes far from simple. This decision requires not only an in depth understanding of the evidence but also the applicability of this evidence to the individual patient considering the anatomic characteristics of the disease, the clinical context, the patient's preferences, social circumstances, and available resources [ie. local expertise and access to PCI and/or CABG]. Furthermore, because there has been evolution of all of these three approaches, interpretation of the evidence has become quite complex. Comparison of different modes of therapy (eg CABG versus medical therapy or CABG to balloon angioplasty) in the past may not be as relevant in the current clinical milieu.

3.1. Advances in medical therapy

Medical therapy has made remarkable advances from a time when patients may have been treated with nitrates alone to contemporary use of a combination of antiplatelets, lipid lowering therapy (statins), beta-blockers (BB) and Angiotensin Converting Enzyme- inhibitors

(ACEI)/Angiotensin Receptor Blocker (ARB). This combined therapy addresses not only patient symptoms but also modifies the disease process such that prognosis is vastly improved [7]. The growth in our understanding the impact of lifestyle modification has also played a central role in how we manage patients with CAD [8].

3.2. Changing clinical patient profile

Due to advances in medical therapy, patients that are now considered for revascularization are also older and have accrued more co-morbidities [9]. These co-morbidities render the interpretation of relevant symptoms more difficult. For example, in a diabetic patient with chronic obstructive lung disease (COPD), it may be difficult to distinguish between dyspnea as an anginal equivalent versus that caused by the underlying pulmonary pathology. The severity of the patients' COPD may also complicate the eligibility for CABG as a mode of revascularization [10, 11]. In fact, in a recent clinical trial comparing CABG versus PCI in complex CAD, significant burden of co-morbidities was the most common reason that patients were felt not to be suitable for CABG and hence entered into the PCI registry [9].

3.3. Advances in angioplasty

Angioplasty has significantly evolved over the last several decades with respect to four principle areas. First, operator training has advanced from informal training courses to 1-2 year formal clinical fellowships [12, 13]. Second, the equipment to perform PCI has significantly improved from plain old balloon angioplasty (POBA) to second-generation drug-eluting stents (DES) and supporting devices to improve PCI outcomes (filter wires, thrombectomy in ST elevation acute coronary syndrome (STEACS), and rotational arthrectomy) [14, 15]. Third, vascular access has evolved from brachial cut-downs with large caliber sheaths (7-8 FR) to increasingly common radial access with smaller caliber sheaths (5 and 6 FR) [5, 15-18]. Finally, concomitant medications have become more sophisticated, from Aspirin (ASA) alone to combination antiplatelets resulting in reduced stent thrombosis [19]. Restenosis has remained in the forefront of limitation to PCI[20]. However, the challenges with restenosis have been significantly reduced with advancement in DES technology [21-23]. Concerns with the thrombosis rates in the setting of discontinuation of dual antiplatelet therapy (DAPT) after DES have been addressed by second-generation DES, which have dramatically reduced this clinical problem [24]. These advances have been paralleled by an increasing use in complex coronary artery disease including left main (LM) disease[25].

3.4. Advances in surgical techniques

From the standpoint of CABG, we have over the years learned the benefits of arterial grafting with the internal mammary artery (IMA) in improving survival [26]. A high long-term patency rate of left internal mammary artery (LIMA) after revascularization of the LAD is well established and is estimated at 88 percent at 10 to 15 years [26]. More recently, to circumvent particular risks associated with sternotomy, there has been some investigation of revascularization of the LAD with the LIMA using a minimally invasive direct coronary artery bypass (MIDCAB) technique [26]. In the setting of multivessel disease (MVD), there has been some discussion of a hybrid approach with MIDCAB for the LAD and PCI of the other vessels. However, the evidence supporting this approach is still limited; the most recent European Society of Cardiology (ESC) Guidelines give a *Class IIb recommendation* to this approach *(Level of Evidence B) for those "patients with conditions likely to prevent healing after sternotomy"* [26]. This approach does have significant promise and further research is required before it is adopted on a population level.

3.5. Evidence of survival benefit for revascularization in stable ischemic heart disease (SIHD)

The current framework for patient selection in treatment strategy for MVD is largely shaped by early studies comparing medical therapy and CABG. This body of evidence has been best synthesized by a meta-analysis performed by Yusuf et al in the Lancet in 1994 [27]. This meta-analysis was an individual patient data analysis of 2549 patients derived from three large randomized controlled trials, the Coronary Artery Surgery Study (CASS), Veterans Administration (VA) study and the European Coronary Surgery Study (ECSS) as well as four other smaller randomized studies [27]. The population studied consisted of patients with stable symptomatic coronary artery disease of a wide spectrum of severity [27]. However, only 10 percent were single vessel disease (1VD); the remainder consisted of MVD with 59.4% affecting the proximal LAD [27].

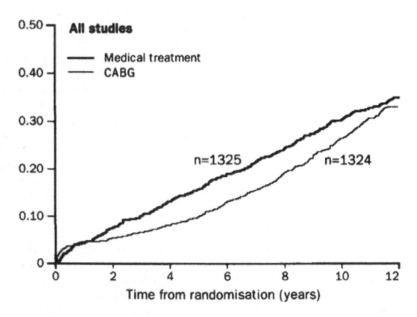

Figure 1. Survival curve for medical therapy versus coronary artery bypass grafting (CABG). Reproduced with permission from Yusuf S. et al. Lancet 1994. 344;8922:563-568

There was an overall statistically significant survival benefit with an **absolute risk reduction (ARR) 5.6% at 5 years, 5.9% at 7 years and 4.1% at 10 years** [Figure 1] [27]. This was likely an overall underestimate of the total treatment effect as there was a 36.4% cross over from the medical group to CABG over that time period whereas 93.7% of those assigned to the surgical group underwent CABG [27]. Subgroup analysis revealed that benefit was largely in those that had *three-vessel disease (3VD) and those with involvement of the proximal LAD* with each of those groups demonstrating a 42% relative risk reduction (RRR) in mortality [27]. In contrast, revascularization in two-vessel disease (2VD) in the absence of involvement of the proximal LAD did not result in a significant mortality benefit [27]. Randomized data is fairly consistent with that of registry data, demonstrating survival benefit for revascularization over medical therapy in those with 3VD; its support for benefit in those with 2VD even in those with proximal left anterior descending (LAD) involvement was non-significant [28]. The latter may be related to improvements in medical therapy.

4. Changing landscape in the treatment of CAD

Many of the earlier studies comparing surgical revascularization with medical therapy was during a period in cardiology where the BB and nitrates were the mainstay of medical therapy. Although antiplatelets were available, these were only taken by approximately 20% of the patients at the time [27]. It may hence be important to interpret these results in the context of current medical practice, which include contemporary treatments (standard secondary prevention with antiplatelets, statin therapy, BB and ACEi) that have all made further advancements in the survival and prognosis of patients with CAD [7].

ASA for secondary prevention has an estimated RRR of 18 percent in total serious vascular events (including stroke and major coronary event) with an **annual ARR of 1.5 percent**; the decrease in major coronary event (non-fatal myocardial infarction (MI) and cardiovascular death) is estimated at **annual ARR of 1.0 percent** [29]. As an adjunctive antiplatelet clopidogrel has further reduced death from cardiovascular causes, non-fatal MI and stroke in patients with Non ST elevation acute coronary syndromes (NSTEACS) with an **ARR of 2.1 percent** [30]. Most recently, newer agents such as prasugrel and ticagralor have both shown benefit compared to clopidogrel in patients with acute coronary syndromes (ACS). Prasugrel compared with clopidogrel in PCI treated ACS has demonstrated an **ARR of 2.2 percent** with regards to death from cardiovascular causes, nonfatal MI or non-fatal stroke over the 6-15 month follow up period [31]. Ticagralor has shown similar reduction in the same composite endpoint in patients with ACS over clopidogrel with an **ARR of 1.9 percent** [32]. In addition, ticagralor also showed an overall **reduction in all cause mortality with an ARR of 1.4 percent** [32].

BB's have a longstanding history in the management of CAD [7]. Although BB's can be used in patients post-MI with a normal ejection fraction (EF), the evidence for this is not as strong as that for those with significant Left Ventricular (LV) dysfunction [8]. It was previously shown that Carvedilol compared with placebo in patients with chronic heart failure (HF) and severe LV dysfunction (average EF 22-23 percent) **reduces all cause mortality with an ARR of 4.6 percent** [33].

The introduction of 3-hydroxyl-3-methyl-glutaryl-coenzyme A (HMG-CoA) reductase inhibitors otherwise known as the "statins," has significantly improved the care of patients with coronary artery disease [34, 35]. Simvastatin 40mg orally daily compared to placebo in patients with known vascular disease was shown in the Heart Protection Study (HPS) to *reduce all cause mortality with an ARR of 1.8 percent* over a five year period [34]. This was paralleled with a **reduction of coronary death with an ARR 1.2%** [34].

ACEi's have also been established to have a significant benefit towards long-term cardiovascular outcomes. It was shown in the Heart Outcomes Prevention Evaluation Study that in high-risk patients (vascular disease or diabetes plus one other risk factor) Ramipril compared with Placebo provides a *relative risk reduction* in myocardial infarction, stroke and death from cardiovascular causes of *21 percent* and *ARR of 3.8 percent* [36] over the mean follow up period of 5 years. There was also a *reduction in all cause death with an ARR of 1.8 percent* [36].

Concurrently, there was the advent and evolution of percutaneous approaches to revascularization. The first generation of angioplasty that truly adopted popular practice involved serial balloon inflations at the site of stenoses restore normal flow dynamics down the conducting epicardial vessels [6]. This approach, although promising was limited by a high rate of restenoses as a result of localized vascular recoil and epithelial hyperplasia [20, 37]. The bare metal stents (BMS) were created as a scaffolding technique that limited the degree of recoil but still faced significant re-stenosis rates due to mediated by injury to the medial layer, increased inflammation resulting from stent strut penetration into the lipid core and ultimately neointimal growth [38].

Pacitaxel and Sirolimus DES were developed in the next phase to overcome the challenge of restenosis requiring repeat intervention [20]. Although there was no difference in mortality or rates of myocardial infarction seen with DES compared with BMS, there were considerable reductions in restenosis rates with an estimated RRR of 0.44 [21, 22, 39-41].

Early enthusiasm for the use of drug eluting stents was curbed by a significantly higher rate of stent thrombosis, particularly in the face of an initially shorter duration (6 months) of dual antiplatelet therapy (DAPT) [22, 42, 43]. Currently the American College of Cardiology/ American Heart Association (ACC/AHA) recommends at least *12 months of DAPT* in patients receiving DES for non-ACS indication and *12 months of DAPT* for ACS indication regardless of the stent type (BMS or DES) *(Class I recommendation, Level B evidence)* [14].

The most recent development in stent technology has been the introduction of second-generation (everolimus and zotarolimus) drug eluting stents. A large Swedish registry observational study containing 94, 384 patients demonstrated the advantage of the second-generation stents over its predecessors (first generation DES and BMS) both in terms of *restenosis* and *definite stent thrombosis* [44]. The second generation DES in this study was shown to have lower risk of restenosis compared with both BMS and the first generation DES with **Hazard Ratios (HR)** of **[0.29, 95% confidence interval (CI) 0.25-0.33]** and **[0.62, CI: 0.53 -0.72]** respectively [44]. The Cobalt Chromium Everolimus eluting stents (CoCr EES) have shown the most promise in reducing stent thrombosis. In a recent network meta-analysis of 50844 patients, the CoCr EES was shown to have a lower rate of 1 year definite stent thrombosis compared to both paclitaxel DES and sirolimus DES with odds ratio (OR) of **[0.41 95% CI 0.24-0.70]** and **[0.28 95% CI 0.16-0.48]** respectively [24]. The CoCr EES also had a lower rate of definite stent thrombosis compared with BMS at 1 year and 2 years with an odds ratio [OR] of

[0.23 95% CI 0.13-0.41) and [0.35, 95% CI 0.17-0.69] respectively [24]. Finally, compared to even the zotarolimus second generation DES, the CoCr EES still demonstrated a robust reduction in stent thrombosis with an OR [0.21, 95% CI 0.17-0.69] at one year [24].

5. PCI versus CABG in SIHD

There have been numerous randomized studies comparing PCI with surgical revascularization in MVD. A recent systematic review including 10 major trials over and the individual data from over 7800 patients found similar mortality in patients treated with CABG (15%) compared to patients treated with angioplasty (16%) over median survival of 5.9 years (p=0.12) [45]. There was, however a significantly lower rate of death or repeat revascularization in those treated with CABG (9.9%) compared with those treated with PCI (24.5%) [45]. This suggests that in fact the major benefit seen in CABG over PCI in this comparison is a lower need for repeat revascularization and is paralleled by a lower incidence of angina in the CABG group (14%) compared to the PCI group (26%) at one year (p<0.0001) [45]. The major caveat to this data is that stenting (which is known to reduce restenosis rates) only represented 37 percent of the total angioplasty group [45].

Subgroup analysis revealed that patients with diabetes have overall *better survival* when treated with surgical revascularization than when treated with angioplasty **with an ARR of 7.7% over 5 years** [45]. More definitive data supporting the use of CABG in patients with diabetes will be presented in *Section 6.2*. Interestingly, there was also a graded age interaction that was significant (p=0.002) [45]. For patients younger than 55 years of age, mortality was lower with PCI (8%) than CABG (10%). In patients between ages 55-64, PCI and CABG had similar mortality rates at 15 and 14 percent respectively [45]. And for patients older than 65 years of age, CABG had a lower overall mortality (20%) compared with PCI (24%) [45]. Prior to this study, this interaction had not been previously reported and we can only speculate whether the effect is a true function of age.

Other subgroups did not prove to contribute any significant interaction to the overall treatment effect [45]. Six of the trials included had POBA as the main mode of PCI whereas four trials used BMS; neither of these groups had significantly different survival rates when compared with surgery [45]. There was no overall interaction contributed by the presence/absence of proximal LAD disease, 3VD, abnormal LV function, previous MI or unstable symptoms [45].

6. Factors favoring surgery as the mode of revascularization

6.1. LV dysfunction

LV function has never been shown to have a significant interaction with mode of revascularization (PCI versus CABG) with regard to survival. In fact, the majority of studies comparing PCI with CABG enrolled a low percentage of patients with abnormal LV function (*20 percent or less*) [45]. However, it has been considered an important variable that favors revascularization with surgery due to historical data showing that patients with significant LV dysfunction have improved survival with CABG compared to medical therapy. An initial signal for preferential benefit of revascularization in patients with mild to moderate LV dysfunction (*LV EF of 35-49%*) was seen in subgroup analyses of the CASS randomized study and the VA study [46, 47]. This was further supported by a meta-analysis demonstrating a significantly longer survival time in 10-year follow up with surgical revascularization over medical therapy in patients with LV dysfunction [10.6 months] compared with those with normal LV function [2.3 months] [27]. These studies however did not address whether a similar effect would be seen in severe LV dysfunction.

The Surgical Treatment for Ischemic Heart Failure (STITCH) trial published recently in 2011, designed to address this question in a randomized comparison of medical therapy versus surgical revascularization in patients with an *EF of 35 percent or less [48]*. There was a non-statistically significant trend (p=0.12) towards decreased all-cause mortality in the surgical group with an relative reduction of 24% and an ARR of 5 percent over the six year follow up period [48]. The lack of statistical significance, in the context of intention to treat analysis, may be related to the disproportionate crossover rate with 17 percent of the patients assigned to medical therapy ultimately receiving coronary bypass surgery [48]. Nevertheless, there was still a significant relative reduction of death from cardiovascular causes of 19 percent (p=0.05) and a significant relative reduction in death from any cause and hospitalization from cardio-vascular causes of 26 percent (p<0.001)[48].

It is unclear why surgical revascularization confers clear benefit in mild to moderate LV dysfunction, and only modest benefit severe LV dysfunction, but there are possible explana-tions. Medical therapy has advanced tremendously since the initial comparisons between medical therapy and surgery, which may decrease the relative mortality benefit between the two treatments during this more contemporary comparison. One could also hypothesize that the beneficial effect of revascularization plateaus at the extremes of LV dysfunction due to irreversible remodelling and/or the progressive increase in associated procedural risk.

There is currently limited data in how revascularization with PCI would affect prognosis in the setting of LV dysfunction[14]. As a result, the most recent ACC/AHA guidelines still recommend CABG for patients with LV EF 35-50 percent with a *IIa recommendation (Grade B evidence)* and a *IIb recommendation (Grade B evidence)* for those with a LV EF of less than 35 percent [49]. And currently, the ACC/AHA guidelines state that there is *insufficient data* to make a recommendation for revascularization with PCI in patients with LV dysfunction [49]. In practice however, if a patient does require revascularization but is not a surgical candidate, that natural decision is that if percutaneous intervention is feasible, that option should be entertained.

6.2. Diabetes favoring surgical revascularization

The Bypass Angioplasty Revascularization Investigation (BARI) was one of the first major landmark studies comparing angioplasty versus coronary bypass in patients with both stable anginal symptoms and unstable angina with MVD. Although there was no significant difference between the two treatments in the overall survival, patients with diabetes tended to have a significantly lower mortality rate with CABG (19.4%) compared with angioplasty (34.5%) with an **ARR of 15.1%** [50]. This finding was further confirmed with a meta-analysis comparing angioplasty with CABG in MVD, albeit with a smaller ARR of 7.7% [45]. In contrast, in non-diabetics there was no overall benefit of surgery over angioplasty[45]. This relationship was corroborated by significant interaction found for the diabetic subgroup (p=0.014) [45]. The interaction was robust and was present even after excluding the data contributed by BARI and when adjusted for various clinical parameters (age, sex, smoking, hypertension, history of MI, heart failure and 3VD) [45].

One hypothesis that may explain why diabetics may have a better outcome with surgery than angioplasty is that restenosis may be more aggressive in this group of patients [20]. It has been well established that one major drawback of percutaneous coronary intervention is the need for repeat revascularization due to restenosis [20]. While restenosis itself may not incur an increased risk of mortality, the repeat exposure to the inherent risk of intervention may be additive. The need for repeat revascularization was certainly more striking in the earlier trials where POBA was used (54 percent within 5 years for the BARI trial) [50]. There has been considerable improvement to both the techniques and technology of PCI first with the development of BMS and now DES which are intended to reduced restenosis rates have been integrated into common practice. However, even in more contemporary trials such as *Synergy between PCI with Taxus and Cardiac Surgery* (SYNTAX), DES conferred a 13.5% need for revascularization compared with 5.9% in patients treated with CABG over a one-year period [51].

BARI 2D is a contemporary trial evaluating revascularization (both PCI and CABG) with intensive medical therapy for SIHD in diabetic patients. No significant difference emerged overall between the two groups in terms of overall mortality, cardiac death or myocardial infarction over the 5-year follow up period [52]. The mode of revascularization was at the discretion of the treating physician and the burden of disease tended to be higher in the CABG group than the PCI group with a mean number of lesions being 5.6 versus 4.3 respectively [52]. Although not specifically designed to compare PCI and CABG as a mode of revascularization, it is still noteworthy that there was a significant difference in death and MI for those revascularized with CABG compared to medical therapy (21.1% versus 29.2% p=0.010); the same comparison in the PCI stratum revealed no difference [52].

To date, the trial most relevant in determining whether the difference between PCI and CABG for revascularizing SIHD in diabetic patients in a randomized fashion is the *FREEDOM* trial [53]. There are 1900 diabetic patients with multivessel disease (defined by >70% stenosis in 2 or more epicardial vessels supplying different vascular territories) that were randomized to CABG versus PCI with DES (Paclitaxel or Sirolimus eluting stent at the discretion of treating physician) with a background of guideline supported optimal medical therapy. The primary endpoint is a composite of all-cause mortality, non-fatal MI or stroke over the mean follow up period of 4.37 years [53]. This consists of a high-risk population with 83% having 3-vessel disease and a significant proportion (32%) requiring insulin therapy [53]. The study results showed that there was a reduction in *primary endpoint all cause death, non-fatal MI and stroke in the CABG group,* with an **ARR of 7.9% (26.6% in the PCI group and 18.7% in the CABG group, p=0.005) and a Number Needed to Treat (NNT) of 12.5 [Figure 2] [53].** There was also a reduction in *all-cause mortality* which was 16.3% in the PCI arm and 10.9% in the CABG arm with an **ARR = 5.4% and NNT of 19 [Figure 2] [53].** This was at the cost of an increase in stroke, as might be expected in the CABG arm of **2.8% Number Needed to Harm (NNH) of 36 [53].**

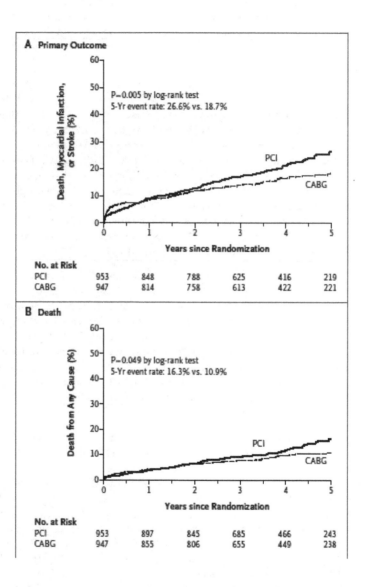

Figure 2. Kaplan-Meier Curves for composite primary outcome (all cause death, non-fatal myocardial infarction or stroke) and all cause death in a comparison between PCI with DES compared with CABG for multivessel disease in diabetic patients. Reproduced with permission from Farkough ME et al. NEJM 2012. DOI 10.1056/NEJMoa1211585.

6.3. Degree of ischemia and revascularization: Is the effect independent of symptoms?

Although there is paucity of randomized data addressing the question of how the degree of functional ischemia relates to the benefit of revascularization, there is observational data that suggests a strong relationship [54, 55]. Adjusted risk models have suggested that patients with *less than a 10-12.5% threshold* of ischemia as demonstrated by stress myocardial perfusion imaging, the survival profile of those treated with medical therapy were similar or even perhaps slightly better than those who are treated with revascularization [54]. However *above the threshold of 10-12.5% of ischemia*, there was a graded incremental survival benefit of revascularization over medical therapy, with a risk adjusted relative risk reduction of 50% [Figure 3] [54].

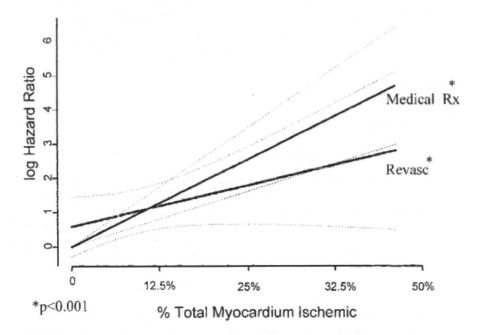

Figure 3. Log hazard ratio for revascularization (Revasc) versus medical therapy (Medical Rx) as a function of % myocardium ischemia based on final cox proportional hazards model. Model, P< 0.0001; interaction, P=0.0305 (Reproduced with permission from Hachamovitch et al. Circulation 2003. 107: 2900-2906).

This data was further corroborated by another observational study demonstrating a similar effect in a group of asymptomatic diabetic patients [55]. This study found a *14% survival benefit* in patients with a high-risk myocardial perfusion scan treated with CABG over medical therapy [55]. Patients treated with PCI in the high-risk scan group did not achieve a survival benefit over medical therapy [55]. This may be due to the fact that, this treatment group consisted of only 10.7% three vessel disease and no patients with left main disease whereas in the CABG group, this was 52.1% and 20.8% respectively [55]. The other caveat to this data is the low overall use of optimal medical therapy, which may overestimate the effect size of revascularization in some anatomic subgroups. The use of ASA, ACEi's and BB's were all 40% or less with no mention of statin therapy [55].

In summary, patients with moderate to high-risk scans by myocardial perfusion have significant survival advantage if treated with revascularization over medical therapy alone *even in the absence of symptoms* [54, 55]. This benefit has more convincingly been demonstrated in patients undergoing CABG [54, 55]. Although the current standard and use of optimal medical therapy has improved over time, this effect is likely still significant. This survival benefit in the high-risk scans has not been clearly demonstrated in patients treated with PCI in stable coronary disease. Recently, the COURAGE trial involving over 2000 patients, which compared optimal medical therapy plus PCI with optimal medical therapy alone in stable CAD included a high prevalence of MVD (over two thirds) associated with the same proportion of multiple reversible defects by myocardial perfusion imaging [56]. This study showed, after exclusion of patients with high-risk anatomy (LM) and markedly positive exercise stress testing (substantial ST depression or hypotensive response in stage I Bruce protocol), no significant difference in all cause death and non-fatal myocardial infarction between the medical therapy and PCI groups [56].

6.4. Impact of complexity of disease

6.4.1. The synergy between PCI with taxus and cardiac surgery (SYNTAX) score

The SYNTAX score was designed as a comprehensive tool to classify the anatomic complexity and functional severity of a patients' coronary anatomy [57]. It is in fact an amalgamation of five different scoring/classification systems which can be distilled into three basic guiding principles: the first which describes the segments of the coronary artery tree; the second which describes the relative importance of the lesion based on the location and vascular territory to which the lesion impedes flow; the third which describes the complexity of the lesion [Table 1].

6.4.2. The SYNTAX trial

As techniques and technology for percutaneous coronary intervention have evolved, there has been an increasing number of patients with multivessel disease treated with percutaneous intervention [58]. The SYNTAX trial has evaluated the PCI versus CABG in patients with highly complex disease in the contemporary context of paclitaxel drug eluting stenting [51]. At 12 months there was a significantly lower incidence of the primary outcome of major cardiac and cerebrovascular events (MACCE) (ie. all cause death, stroke myocardial infarction or repeat revascularization) CABG group compared than the PCI group with an **ARR of 5.4% or NNT 19** [51]. This was largely driven by an increase need for repeat revascularization as the rates of *all cause death, MI or stroke was similar between the two groups* [51]. In the initial subgroup analysis at 12 months, while there was a trend towards lower MACCE in the CABG group compared to the PCI group as the SYNTAX scores increased, a significantly lower rate of the primary outcome could only be demonstrated at the highest SYNTAX scores (>33) [Figure 4] [51].

Principle	Description
Definition and segmentation of the coronary artery tree	1. The coronary tree can be divided into 16 major segments
Functional significance	2. Functional importance of the particular epicardial vessel is weighted according to the percentage of the left ventricle to which it supplies. For example the left main supplies 5 times the vascular territory compared to that of a dominant RCA; hence the LM will be given a score of 5 whereas the RCA will be given a score of 1.
Lesion Complexity	3. The complexity of the lesion itself can be described in terms of
	a. Degree of involvement of side branches, anatomic configuration of lesions
	b. Presence or absence of a total occlusions and presence of collaterals
	c. Lesion length
	d. Tortuousity of vessel
	e. Presence or absence of heavy calcification
	f. Presence or absence of Thrombus
	g. Presence or absence of diffuse disease

Table 1. Principles underlying the development of the SYNTAX score

The 3-year follow-up for this study more definitively demonstrated that PCI and CABG tended to have similar cardiovascular outcomes in patients with lower complexity while at higher levels of anatomical complexity, patients that underwent CABG faired better [Figure 5] [59]. At three-year follow-up, patients with 3VD in the CABG group versus the PCI group with intermediate complexity (SYNTAX Score 23-32) had overall **decrease in MI with an ARR of 5.8%** and those with the highest complexity (SYNTAX Score >33) had a decrease in **all cause mortality (ARR of 6.6%) and a decrease in MI (ARR of 5.3%)** [51, 59]. This was also reflected in an *overall lower all-cause death* in the 3VD patients treated with CABG versus PCI with an *ARR of 3.8% (p=0.02)* and a *lower rate of cardiac death* in those treated with CABG versus PCI *ARR 3.3% (p=0.01)* [59]. Interestingly, there was no significant difference for all-cause death or cardiac death between the CABG group versus the PCI group among patients with LM disease [59]. In contrast to those with 3VD, there were only significantly lower MACCE rates among patients with LM disease treated with CABG compared with PCI at the highest SYNTAX scores (>33) [59]. Although it is difficult to make precise conclusions regarding the subgroup analyses, the overall trends are certainly compelling.

The recent SYNTAX trial has heralded a new era in revascularization. The recent European Guidelines have responded to the findings by giving a **IIa recommendation (level B evidence)** to PCI for revascularization in 3VD with low angiographic complexity (SYNTAX score ≤22) while giving a **class III recommendation (level A evidence)** for revascularization of such patients moderate to high angiographic complexity (SYNTAX score >22) [26]. The most recent ACC/AHA PCI guidelines state that in patients with 3VD with or without proximal LAD, revascularization with PCI for the purposes of prognosis is of **uncertain benefit (IIb recommendation, level B evidence)** [14]. In these populations, CABG is still given **Class I recommendation (level B evidence)** [Table 2 and 3] [14, 26].

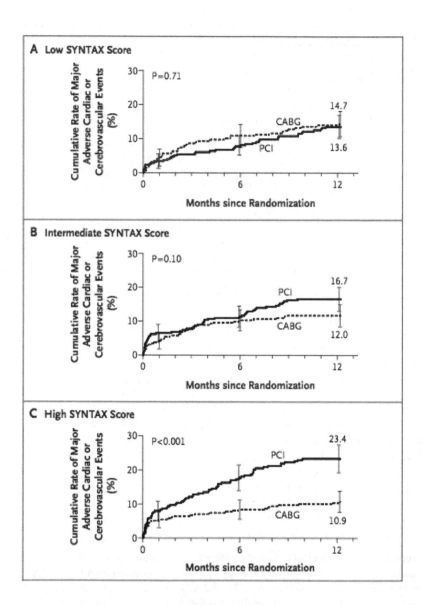

Figure 4. 12-month Subgroup analysis of the rates of (all cause death, stroke, myocardial infarction and repeat revascularization) between those treated by CABG versus PCI stratified by SYNTAX score. A significant difference in the overall rates was not significantly different at low (<22) and intermediate (23-32) SYNTAX scores. At the highest SYNTAX score (>33), there was a significantly lower rate of major cardiac and cerebrovascular events. Reproduced with permission from Serruys PW et al. NEJM 2009. 360;10: 961-972.

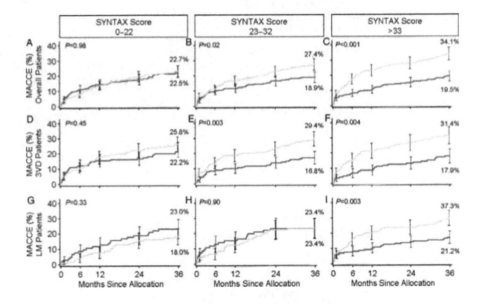

Figure 5. 3-year subgroup analysis of the rates of MACCE (all cause death, stroke, myocardial infarction and repeat revascularization) between those treated by CABG (blue line) versus PCI (yellow line) stratified by SYNTAX score: Low SYNTAX Score (0-22), Intermediate SYNTAX Score (23-32), High SYNTAX Score (>33). Results are provided for overall group (A-C), 3VD patients (D-F) and LM patients (G-I). Reproduced with permission from Kappetein et al. European Heart Journal 2011. 32: 2125-2134.

Subset of CAD by anatomy	Favours CABG	Favours PCI
1VD or 2VD - non-proximal LAD	IIb C	I C
1VD or 2VD - proximal LAD	I A	IIa B
3VD simple lesions, full functional revascularization achievable with PCI, SYNTAX score ≤22	I A	IIa B
3VD complex lesions, incomplete revascularization achievable with PCI, SYNTAX score >22	I A	III A
Left main (isolated or 1VD, ostium/shaft)	I A	IIa B
Left main (isolated or 1VD, distal bifurcation)	I A	IIb B
Left main + 2VD or 3VD, SYNTAX score ≤32	I A	IIb B
Left main + 2VD or 3VD, SYNTAX score ≥33	I A	III B

Table 2. ESC Guidelines on revascularization for complex coronary disease. Indications for CABG and PCI are tabulated for stable patients with low predicted surgical mortality and lesions suitable for either modes of revascularization. CABG= coronary artery bypass grafting; CAD= coronary artery disease; LAD = left anterior descending; PCI= percutaneous coronary intervention; VD= vessel disease. Reproduced with permission from Wijns W et al. European Heart Journal 2010. 31: 2501-2555.

Anatomical Setting	Class of Recommendation	Level of Evidence
UPLM or complex CAD		
CABG and PCI	I—Heart Team approach recommended	C
CABG and PCI	IIa—Calculation of STS and SYNTAX scores	B
UPLM*		
CABG	I	B
PCI	IIa—For SHD when both of the following are present • Anatomic conditions associated with a low risk of PCI procedural complications and a high likelihood of good long-term outcome (eg, a low SYNTAX score of ≤22, ostial or trunk left main CAD) • Clinical characteristics that predict a significantly increased risk of adverse surgical outcomes (eg, STS-predicted risk of operative mortality ≥5%)	B
	IIa—For UA/NSTEMI if not a CABG candidate	B
	IIa—For STEMI when distal coronary flow is TIMI flow grade <3 and PCI can be performed more rapidly and safely than CABG	C
	IIb—For SIHD when both of the following are present • Anatomic conditions associated with a low to intermediate risk of PCI procedural complications and an intermediate to high likelihood of good long-term outcome (eg, low-intermediate SYNTAX score of <33, bifurcation left main CAD) • Clinical characteristics that predict an increased risk of adverse surgical outcomes (eg, moderate-severe COPD, disability from prior stroke, or prior cardiac surgery; STS-predicted risk of operative mortality >2%)	B
	III: Harm—For SIHD in patients (versus performing CABG) with unfavorable anatomy for PCI and who are good candidates for CABG	B
3-vessel disease with or without proximal LAD artery disease*		
CABG	I	B
	IIa—It is reasonable to choose CABG over PCI in patients with complex 3-vessel CAD (eg, SYNTAX score >22) who are good candidates for CABG	B
PCI	IIb—Of uncertain benefit	B
2-vessel disease with proximal LAD artery disease*		
CABG	I	B
PCI	IIb—Of uncertain benefit	B
2-vessel disease without proximal LAD artery disease*		
CABG	IIa—With extensive ischemia	B
	IIb—Of uncertain benefit without extensive ischemia	C
PCI	IIb—Of uncertain benefit	B
1-vessel proximal LAD artery disease		
CABG	IIa—With LIMA for long-term benefit	B
PCI	IIb—Of uncertain benefit	B
1-vessel disease without proximal LAD artery involvement		
CABG	III: Harm	B
PCI	III: Harm	B
LV dysfunction		
CABG	IIa—EF 35% to 50%	B
CABG	IIb—EF <35% without significant left main CAD	B
PCI	Insufficient data	
Survivors of sudden cardiac death with presumed ischemia-mediated VT		
CABG	I	B
PCI	I	C
No anatomic or physiologic criteria for revascularization		
CABG	III: Harm	B
PCI	III: Harm	B

Table 3. ACC Guidelines on revascularization for complex coronary disease to improve survival. Indications for CABG and PCI are tabulated. CABG = coronary artery bypass grafting; COPD= chronic obstructive pulmonary disease; EF= ejection fraction; LAD=left anterior descending artery; LIMA= left internal mammary artery; LV =left ventricular; N/A= not applicable; PCI = percutaneous coronary intervention; SIHD = stable ischemic heart disease; STEMI= ST-elevation myocardial infarction; STS= Society of Thoracic Surgeons; SYNTAX = Synergy between percutaneous coronary intervention with TAXUS and Cardiac Surgery; TIMI= Thrombolysis in myocardial infarction; UA/NSTEMI =unstable angina/ non-ST elevation myocardial infarction; UPLM= unprotected left main disease; VT=ventricular tachycardia. Reproduced with permission from Levine GN et al. Circulation 2011. 124: e574-e651.

For those with unprotected left main disease (UPLM), both the ACC and ESC guidelines still give a **Class I** *recommendation for CABG in all cases* **(Classified as Grade A evidence for ESC and Grade B evidence for ACC)** [14, 26]. They have both also given a **IIa recommendation for PCI in Stable Ischemic Heart Disease (SIHD) in UPLM when the SYNTAX is 22 or less (eg isolated ostial or main trunk LM) and IIb recommendation for PCI for low or intermediate SYNTAX score (<33) (Level B evidence)** [14, 26]

It is recognized however, that some populations are not expected to derive prognostic benefit from revascularization. In such groups for the purposes of alleviating symptoms refractory to optimal medical therapy, CABG and PCI have equivalent **Class I recommendation (level A evidence) unless SYNTAX is >22 in which case CABG is still favored (Class IIa recommendation, level B evidence)** [14].

7. PCI versus CABG in acute coronary syndromes versus stable ischemic coronary artery disease

7.1. Non-ST-elevation acute coronary syndromes (NSTEACS)

Although there are limited studies designed to address this specific question, it is generally accepted that the same considerations that are used to decide between PCI and CABG in stable ischemic coronary artery disease would be applied when faced with an NSTEACS **(Class I recommendation, Level B evidence)** [14]. Comparisons between PCI and CABG have typically included a mixture of patients with stable and unstable symptoms [45]. The ERACI II study contained the highest proportion of patients with unstable symptoms constituting 92% of the randomized patients whereas MASS II included the least with 0% having unstable symptoms [60, 61]. However in a large meta-analysis including individual patient data from 10 large randomized studies (n=7812) did not reveal any significant interaction between the presence or absence of unstable symptoms and mode of revascularization (PCI vs CABG) with respect to mortality outcomes over a 5 year period [45].

The optimal approach to PCI in the setting of a NSTEACS and MVD is still somewhat uncertain. There are currently no randomized trials in the literature comparing the multivessel PCI to culprit only PCI in NSTEACS [62].

7.2. ST -elevation acute coronary syndromes (STEACS)

Primary PCI remains the main modality of revascularization in STEACS *(Class I recommendation, Level A evidence)*. It is common to encounter MVD during the index angiogram for STEACS having an estimated incidence of up to 40-50 percent [62]. Current evidence supports primary PCI of the culprit vessel only, in the absence of hemodynamic instability, as the optimal approach [14, 62, 63]. *Multivessel PCI in this setting has been associated with a higher mortality and is not recommended (Class III recommendation, Level B evidence) [14, 62, 63].* The approach to residual coronary disease has been a subject of controversy and the decisions are likely made clinically on an individual basis.

7.3 Cardiogenic shock

The optimal mode of revascularization in patients with multivessel disease and cardiogenic shock is still under debate due to lack of supporting evidence for or against either PCI or CABG. It has been previously shown in the **Should We Emergently Revascularize Occluded Arteries for Cardiogenic Shock (SHOCK) Trial** that urgent revascularization with PCI or CABG for cardiogenic shock in the setting of STEACS has *mortality benefit* with an **ARR of 13 percent** or **NNT of 8** at 6 months compared with medical management [64]. This difference continued out to one year and remained stable at long-term follow up [Figure 6] [65, 66]. In the revascularization group, 64 percent were treated with angioplasty whereas 36 percent were treated with CABG [64]. Interestingly, because the mode of revascularization was at the discretion of the treating physicians, patients treated with CABG compared with those that received PCI tended to more often have LM disease and 3VD [64]. Nevertheless, there was no significant difference between patients treated with PCI versus CABG at either 30 days or at 1 year [64]. Certainly the advantage of PCI for revascularization over CABG would be a reduced time required to achieve revascularization; the time of randomization to first revascularization attempt was 0.9 hour for PCI and 2.7 hours for CABG [64].

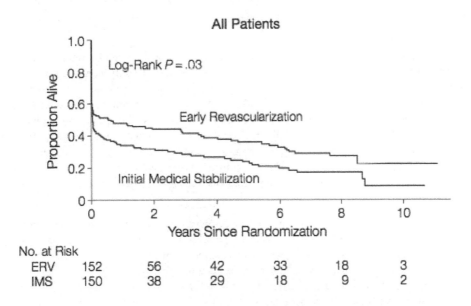

Figure 6. Kaplan-Meier Survival Curves For Early Revascularization Versus Initial Medical Stabilization in Long Term Follow-Up. ERV= Early Revascularization; IMS =Initial Medical Stabilization. Reproduced with permission from Hochman JS. et al. JAMA 2006. 295;21: 2511-2515.

There is a lack of randomized data regarding the optimal mode of revascularization in cardiogenic shock for acute coronary syndromes [67]. Currently, both the ACC and ESC guidelines recommend that PCI (or emergency CABG) should be performed on patients who candidates for revascularization in the setting of STEMI and severe heart failure or cardiogenic shock *(Class I recommendation, Level B evidence)* [14, 26]. Although the data upon which this recommendation is based does not show a preferential benefit to either mode of revascularization, both guidelines favor PCI as the primary mode of revascularization in cardiogenic shock [14, 26]. The ACC guidelines do recognize however, that "select patients with severe 3VD or LM disease can benefit from emergency CABG" [14].

8. Treatment of hemodynamically significant disease

Currently, the ACC/ AHA defines a significant stenosis as "Greater than or equal to 70% luminal diameter narrowing, by visual assessment, of an epicardial stenosis measured in the "worst view" angiographic projection [68]." The exception is the left main artery in which a significant stenosis is defined as " greater or equal to 50% luminal diameter narrowing [68]." A challenge in the interpretation of the data surrounding comparisons of PCI versus CABG the variability in definitions of "significant disease." Interestingly, many of the landmark trials comparing PCI versus CABG actually defined a significant stenosis as greater or equal to 50% [27, 45, 51].

Even in the presence of a significant stenosis, myocardial blood flow can be maintained by compensatory mechanisms at rest [69]. Consequently, hemodynamically significant disease has been defined by those lesions, which produce a reduction in coronary flow reserve under conditions of maximal hyperemia [69, 70]. Reduction of coronary flow reserve is generally observed in lesions with as little as 50 percent stenosis but progressively worsens with the degree of narrowing [70]. There are two implications of this clinically. First, there is a significant interobserver and intraobserver variability in the degree of angiographic stenosis [69]. Second, the hemodynamic significance of a given lesion is dependent on the severity of the stenosis, the length of the lesion as well as the presence of collateral blood flow [71].

Aims to quantify the functional significance of coronary stenosis lead to the development of the concept Fractional Flow Reserve (FFR) [72]. FFR is a hemodynamic construct defined as the maximal blood flow distal to a stenosis compared with the maximal blood flow in the same vessel, hypothetically in the absence of any stenosis, conditions of maximal hyperemia [72]. Flow can be characterized by the following equation: Pressure (P) = Flow (Q) * Resistance (R) [72]. For a given lesion, the FFR is the maximal flow for the stenotic vessel (Qs)/ maximal flow if the vessel were normal (Qn). Since, under maximal hyperemia, the resistance becomes a constant, Q is only dependent on the pressure and fractional flow reserve can be defined by a ratio of aortic pressure (Pa)/ pressure distal to the lesion (Pd) [Figure 7] [72]. FFR allows for the functional assessment of ischemia at the time of coronary angiogram [72].

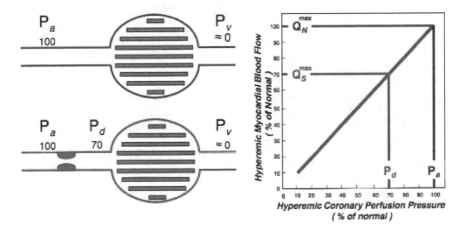

Figure 7. A schematic depiction of the concept of fractional flow reserve. On the right is the graphical correlation between Flow Q and perfusion pressure P under conditions of maximal hyperemia. The maximal blood flow in the stenotic vessel Q_s (Red Lines) is directly proportional to the perfusion pressure distal to the lesion. The maximal blood flow in the same vessel hypothetically without the stenosis Q_N (Blue Lines) is proportional to the perfusion pressure proximal to the stenosis Pa which is the same as aortic pressure. Q_s/Q_N is therefore equal to Pd/Pa. Reproduced with permission from Pijls NHJ et al. JACC 2012. 59: 1045-57.

The use of FFR will be come increasingly more relevant in the assessment of patients with multivessel disease. The **Fractional Flow Reserve Versus Angiography for Multivessel Evaluation (FAME)** was a study randomizing 1005 patients to either angiographically guided PCI or PCI guided by fractional flow reserve in patients with multivessel disease of at least moderate severity (greater or equal to 50%) [73]. Patients in the angiographic group were revascularized if PCI was indicated based on visual assessment of angiographic data and clinical data; patients in the FFR group only had PCI if the FFR was < 0.80 [73]. The combined outcome of death, myocardial infarction and repeat revascularization was significantly less in those treated with FFR guided PCI (18.3%) than the angiographically guided PCI (13.2%) [Figure 8] [73]. Death and myocardial infarction, although not a pre-specified outcome, was also significantly less in the FFR group (11.1%) versus the angiographic group (7.3%) [73]. This difference persisted to the two-year follow-up [74].

Although FFR is early in its development, certainly it has the potential to play a role in classifying the severity of disease for decision-making in MVD. Consider a patient with 3VD with a 50 percent lesion at the proximal LAD. If the proximal LAD lesion is FFR is greater than 0.80, this patient may in fact be classified as two vessel disease with no hemodynamic involvement of the proximal LAD and hence should receive PCI. While there is limited research exploring the use of FFR in determining the mode of revascularization, this is certainly an area worthy of further study. Currently the ACC advocates the use of FFR guiding revascularization decisions in stable ischemic heart disease with moderate lesions with 50-70% stenosis (**IIa recommendation, level A evidence**) [14].

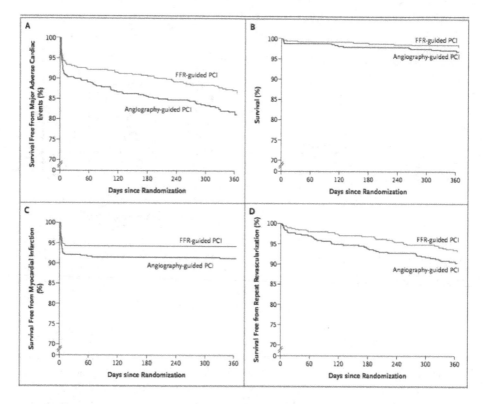

Figure 8. Kaplan-Meier Survival Curves according to study group PCI guided by angiography alone versus PCI guided by FFR in addition to angiography. FFR=fractional flow reserve, PCI=percutaneous coronary intervention. Reproduced with permission from Tonino PAL et al. Fractional flow reserve versus angiography or guiding percutanous coronary intervention. NEJM 2009. 360(3):213-224.

9. Current trends in PCI versus CABG in North America

The practice patterns regarding PCI and CABG have changed dramatically within the last 10-15 years. In the earlier part of this last decade, rates of PCI have been observed to be on the rise both in the United States and in Canada despite relatively more static rates of CABG over that same period [75, 76]. Furthermore, although there is some signal that the trend in PCI rates have begun to plateau or reverse in the latter part of this decade both in the United states and in Canada, there is still a consistent increase in the overall PCI: CABG ratio [77, 78].

These recent trends have been an area of increasing research interest, as it seems paradoxical in the context of relatively consistent practice guidelines from the ACC and the ESC supporting the use of CABG as the first line mode of revascularization in prognostically important stable

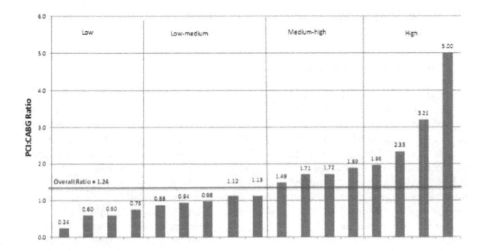

Figure 9. Variation in Revascularization for Multivessel Disease Across 17 Cardiac Centers in Ontario. Reproduced with permission from Schwalm JD et al. SYNTAX Score and Real World Revascularization Patterns. Canadian Cardiovascular Congress 2011 Vancouver, BC. Abstract Presentation.

ischemic coronary artery disease [Figure 9] [14, 26]. In fact, recent data has demonstrated a rise in PCI with DES in patients with Class I recommendation for surgery [25].

Significant variability in PCI:CABG ratio between provinces/states, between hospitals and even between individual interventionalists suggests that the trends in revascularization practices are not entirely explained by changes in population or advancements in revascularization techniques [76-80]. In Ontario, Canada, PCI to CABG ratios vary considerably between hospitals from 1.3 to 6.1 [81]. In multivessel disease, this ratio ranges from 0.24 to 5.0 [figure 9] [82]. The physician performing the diagnostic catheterization (interventional cardiologist versus non-interventional cardiologist), the coronary anatomy (LM, 3VD, 2VD), and the treating hospital were the three strongest determinants of the ultimate therapeutic strategy [58].

Two possible hypotheses for the presence of such dramatic variability in the management of multi-vessel disease include misinterpretation of the evidence and misclassification of disease complexity at the time of diagnostic angiogram. There are complex interacting variables upon which the final therapeutic decision is based, including: (1) complexity of coronary anatomy, (2) presence or absence of prognostically important factors favoring surgery, (3) degree of active functional ischemia, (4) complex co-morbid state of patient, (5) patient preferences and social factors, (6) local resources and expertise. All of these factors may affect the patient's suitability for CABG and likelihood to benefit prognostically from surgical revascularization. Application of the large body of evidence in this variable clinical milieu is a complex process. The management algorithm is further complicated when considering the patient's role in the decision-making process and the steps required to ensure truly "informed" patient consent.

10. Angioplasty versus bypass surgery: An evolving complex decision analysis

10.1. Establishing a general approach

Decisions regarding revascularization are complex and have been founded on decades of evidence. This body of evidence has evolved in parallel with advances in treatment but also a patient population with increasing medical complexity. Therefore, a contemporary approach to MVD and revascularization must be founded on an understanding of the wide spectrum of disease severity, advances in medical/surgical therapy, diversity in patient populations, patient preference and social circumstances. Optimal treatment strategies must apply the most current evidence in an appropriate clinical context. Furthermore, guiding principles of management with a multidisciplinary 'Heart Team' approach should be the cornerstone of state of the art treatment of multivessel coronary artery disease as supported by recent revascularization guidelines [14]. The basic approach should address a number of basic clinical questions which address the (1) therapeutic goals of the case, (2) the presence or absence of clinical evidence to support revascularization, (3) the presence/absence of prognostic factors that may make surgical revascularization more favorable, (4) whether the anatomy favor PCI or CABG, (5) is the patient a good surgical candidate should prognostic disease be present, (6) does the patient have any particular preferences and (7) are there ambiguities that would benefit from further discussion by a Heart Team [Table 4].

Fundamental Question	
Therapeutic Goals:	● Can we improve survival? ● Can we improve symptoms? ● Can we improve both?
Clinical Evidence to support revascularization	● Severity of disease ● Severity of Symptoms ● Degree of Ischemia ● Degree of Medical Optimization
Prognostic Factors that may make surgical revascularization more favorable?	LM, 3VD, or 2VD with proximal LAD with ● DM ● LV dysfunction ● High burden of ischemia ("/≥12.5 percent)
Does anatomy favor one mode of revascularization versus the other?	● Surgical targets ● Diffuseness of disease ● Complexity
Is the patient a good surgical candidate?	Consider: ● Age ● Co-morbidities ● Anatomy
Patient Preference and Social Factors	Discussed off the catheterization table
Ambiguities in Case?	Would this benefit from discussion with the Heart Team?

Table 4. Key clinical questions forming the basis of the therapeutic decision for management of multivessel coronary artery disease.

The fundamental basis of our decisions rest on what therapeutic goals can be achieved: *improvement of survival, improvement of symptoms or both*. It is important to make this distinction because although the goal would naturally to improve on both; consider the following two clinical scenarios:

- In a 50 year-old asymptomatic patient with 70% distal LM, CABG is the treatment of choice regardless of his symptom profile because of known survival benefit with surgical revascularization **(Class I, Level A evidence)**[14]

- In a 90 year-old, medically optimized, CCS class III patient who has 3VD and normal ejection fraction, his age may undermine any treatment for the purposes of prognosis, hence PCI may be favored if technically feasible as the overriding goal is for relief of symptoms. **(Class I, Level A evidence)**[14]

If the intent is to improve survival, there is good evidence that supports revascularization in certain patient populations: significant left main (>50%) or 3VD, 2VD with proximal LAD with diabetes LV dysfunction and/or high burden of functional ischemia).

If the intent is primarily to *improve symptoms (eg. The clinical profile undermines the prognostic benefit of surgical revascularization)*, there is good evidence that revascularization with PCI is of benefit in those who are symptomatic despite optimal medical therapy if technically feasible. But with advances in medical therapy, it is reasonable to maximize medical treatment before considering revascularization [56].

10.2. The decision algorithm

Based on existing evidence and guidelines, we have developed an algorithm that may help guide decision-making in the management of MVD [Figure10]. There are a number of factors that support surgical revascularization in SIHD for improving survival over medical therapy or PCI, namely: 1) LM disease, 3VD and likely some subsets of 2VD with proximal LAD; 2) MVD in the presence of mild to moderate LV dysfunction (35-49%) 3) MVD in the presence of diabetes 4) coronary anatomy of intermediate to high level of complexity (SYNTAX >22) and 5) high burden of ischemia (>12.5%). If these are present, then surgery should be considered first unless patient preference dictates otherwise **(Class I recommendation, Level B Evidence).**

If the patient does have prognostic disease, then considering the overall coronary anatomy, patients clinical profile and co-morbidities must be considered to ultimately guide the appropriate therapeutic decision. These factors may alter the likelihood of benefit from revascularization and also affect the patients' potential eligibility CABG and PCI.

If the patient does not appear to have prognostic disease and is not likely to prognostically benefit from revascularization, then the primary goal of treatment would be symptoms. The first goal of alleviating symptoms is medical optimization. If the patient has unacceptable symptoms despite optimal medical therapy, then revascularization (PCI or CABG) would be indicated **(Class I recommendation, Level A Evidence).**

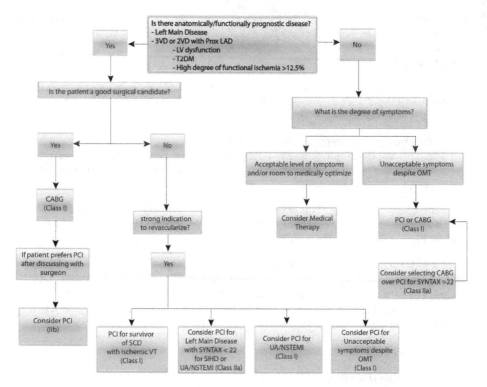

Figure 10. Suggested approach for decision making in multivessel coronary artery disease. CAD= coronary artery disease; CABG= coronary artery bypass grafting; LAD= left anterior descending artery; LM = left main disease; LV= Left Ventricular; OMT= optimal medical therapy; PCI= percutaneous coronary intervention; SCD= sudden cardiac death; SYNTAX = The Synergy between PCI with Taxus and Cardiac Surgery; T2DM= Type 2 Diabetes Mellitus; UA/NSTEMi = unstable angina/Non ST elevation myocardial infarction; VT= ventricular tachycardia; 3VD = Three vessel disease; 2VD = two vessel disease.

11. The Role of the heart team in the future of multivessel disease

The management of CAD with the advances in revascularization techniques and medical therapy, changing patient population and constantly expanding body of knowledge is becoming increasingly more complex. Such complexity would intuitively benefit from a broad spectrum of expertise. There is currently increasing interest in the area of multidisciplinary decision-making and both ACC and ESC have recommended that a Heart Team approach be implemented in the management of UPLM disease or complex CAD *(Class I recommendation, Level C Evidence)* [14, 26]. It is envisioned that with the joint involvement of the interventional cardiologist, the cardiac surgeon and a non-invasive cardiologist, there will be a more balanced, consistent management of these complex cases. From the patient's perspective, this approach would conceivably allow them to be more informed and involved in the ultimate treatment decision. There is currently limited data on the true impact of the Heart Team and this is certainly an area of worthy future research.

12. The future of research in complex coronary artery disease

The approach to the management of complex CAD will continue to change with exponential growth of knowledge in this area. The majority of clinical trials involving CABG and PCI were largely based on complete revascularization of lesions greater than 50 percent [45]. Use of FFR has shown that PCI with DES of moderately severe lesions (50-70 percent) guided by angiography alone compared with PCI of lesions guided by both angiography and hemodynamic significance (FFR< 0.80) may actually confer a higher rate of death and MI [73]. Given our knowledge of this finding, the SYNTAX trial (where the threshold for revascularization was also a stenosis of 50 percent or greater) may conceivably have different results if FFR was used to guide therapy. Furthermore, investigations with the new second-generation DES, a now better understanding of how to utilize FFR and definition of the impact of coronary complexity may serve as a guide to better define the populations that may benefit from PCI versus CABG.

The other area requiring more research is in the arena of collaboration for decision-making in multivessel disease. The Heart Team, although a promising concept would benefit from formal validation. We also need to better define what type of institutions and what type of cases would most benefit from formal evaluation with a Heart Team approach. Furthermore as these decisions become more complex, we will also need to find better methods/mechanisms of informed balanced patient involvement in the final management decision.

Complex CAD remains a challenging area both from the scientific and the clinical point of view. The goal should be to build on the research foundations in the management of MVD CAD thus far and continue to improve our understanding of how to better manage and care for patients with complex CAD.

Abbreviations

ACC	American College of Cardiology
ACEi	Angiotensin Converting Enzyme inhibitor
ARB	Angiotensin Receptor Blocker
AHA	American Heart Association
ARR	Absolute risk reduction
ASA	Aspirin
BB	Beta Blocker
BMS	Bare metal stent

CABG	Coronary artery bypass grafting
CAD	Coronary artery disease
CI	95% Confidence interval
COPD	Chronic obstructive pulmonary disease
DAPT	Dual antiplatelet therapy
DES	Drug eluting stent
ESC	European Society of Cardiology
HMG-CoA	3-hydroxyl-3-methyl-glutaryl-coenzyme A
LAD	Left anterior descending artery
LIMA	Left internal mammary artery
LM	Left main
MID CAB	minimally invasive direct coronary artery bypass
NNH	Number Needed to Harm
NNT	Number Needed to Treat
NSTEACS	Non ST elevation acute coronary syndrome
NSTEMI	Non ST elevation myocardial infarction
PCI	Percutaneous coronary intervention
POBA	Plain old balloon angioplasty
RRR	Relative Risk Reduction
SCD	Sudden cardiac death
SIHD	Stable ischemic heart disease
STEACS	ST elevation acute coronary syndrome
STEMI	ST elevation myocardial infarction
SYNTAX	Synergy between PCI with Taxus and Cardiac Surgery
UA	Unstable angina
UPLM	Unprotected left main disease
VT	Ventricular tachycardia
3VD	Three vessel disease
2VD	Two vessel disease

Author details

Michael Tsang and JD Schwalm

Department of Medicine, Division of Cardiology, McMaster University, Hamilton Health Sciences, Population Health Research Institute, Hamilton, Ontario, Canada

References

[1] Macklem, P.T., *Stephen Hales, an unrecognized giant of medicine.* Osler Libr Newsl, 2010(114): p. 1-4.

[2] Bourassa, M.G., *The history of cardiac catheterization.* Can J Cardiol, 2005. 21(12): p. 1011-4.

[3] Proudfit, W.L., E.K. Shirey, and F.M. Sones, Jr., *Selective cine coronary arteriography. Correlation with clinical findings in 1,000 patients.* Circulation, 1966. 33(6): p. 901-10.

[4] Sones, F.M.J. and E.K. Shirey, *Cine coronary arteriography.* Mod Con Cardiov Dis, 1962. 31: p. 735.

[5] Mueller, R.L. and T.A. Sanborn, *The history of interventional cardiology: cardiac catheterization, angioplasty, and related interventions.* Am Heart J, 1995. 129(1): p. 146-72.

[6] Berry, D., *The unlocking of the coronary arteries: origins of angioplasty. A short historical review of arterial dilatation from Dotter to the creative Gruentzig.* Eur Heart J, 2009. 30(12): p. 1421-2.

[7] Nabel, E.G. and E. Braunwald, *A tale of coronary artery disease and myocardial infarction.* N Engl J Med, 2012. 366(1): p. 54-63.

[8] Smith, S.C., Jr., et al., *AHA/ACCF Secondary Prevention and Risk Reduction Therapy for Patients with Coronary and other Atherosclerotic Vascular Disease: 2011 update: a guideline from the American Heart Association and American College of Cardiology Foundation.* Circulation, 2011. 124(22): p. 2458-73.

[9] Head, S.J., et al., *Risk profile and 3-year outcomes from the SYNTAX percutaneous coronary intervention and coronary artery bypass grafting nested registries.* JACC Cardiovasc Interv, 2012. 5(6): p. 618-25.

[10] Fuster, R.G., et al., *Prognostic value of chronic obstructive pulmonary disease in coronary artery bypass grafting.* Eur J Cardiothorac Surg, 2006. 29(2): p. 202-9.

[11] Ried, M., et al., *Mild-to-moderate COPD as a risk factor for increased 30-day mortality in cardiac surgery.* Thorac Cardiovasc Surg, 2010. 58(7): p. 387-91.

[12] Hirshfeld, J.W., Jr., et al., *American College of Cardiology training statement on recommendations for the structure of an optimal adult interventional cardiology training program: a report of the American College of Cardiology task force on clinical expert consensus documents.* J Am Coll Cardiol, 1999. 34(7): p. 2141-7.

[13] Ryan, T.J., K. F.J., and R. W.A., *Clinical competence in percutaneous transluminal coronary angioplasty. A statement for physicians from the ACP/ACC/AHA Task Force on Clinical Privileges in Cardiology.* Circulation, 1990. 81(6): p. 2041-6.

[14] Levine, G.N., et al., *2011 ACCF/AHA/SCAI Guideline for Percutaneous Coronary Intervention: a report of the American College of Cardiology Foundation/American Heart Associa-*

tion Task Force on Practice Guidelines and the Society for Cardiovascular Angiography and Interventions. Circulation, 2011. 124(23): p. e574-651.

[15] Holmes, D.R., Jr., *Creativity, ingenuity, serendipity.* Can J Cardiol, 2005. 21(12): p. 1061-5.

[16] Campeau, L., *Entry sites for coronary angiography and therapeutic interventions: from the proximal to the distal radial artery.* Can J Cardiol, 2001. 17(3): p. 319-25.

[17] Gruntzig, A.R., A. Senning, and W.E. Siegenthaler, *Nonoperative dilatation of coronary-artery stenosis: percutaneous transluminal coronary angioplasty.* N Engl J Med, 1979. 301(2): p. 61-8.

[18] Molajo, A.O., et al., *Comparison of the performance of superflow (5F) and conventional 8F catheter for cardiac catheterization by the femoral route.* Cathet Cardiovasc Diagn, 1987. 13(4): p. 275-6.

[19] Chhatriwalla, A.K. and D.L. Bhatt, *Should dual antiplatelet therapy after drug-eluting stents be continued for more than 1 year?: Dual antiplatelet therapy after drug-eluting stents should be continued for more than one year and preferably indefinitely.* Circ Cardiovasc Interv, 2008. 1(3): p. 217-25.

[20] Farooq, V., B.D. Gogas, and P.W. Serruys, *Restenosis: delineating the numerous causes of drug-eluting stent restenosis.* Circ Cardiovasc Interv, 2011. 4(2): p. 195-205.

[21] Trikalinos, T.A., et al., *Percutaneous coronary interventions for non-acute coronary artery disease: a quantitative 20-year synopsis and a network meta-analysis.* Lancet, 2009. 373(9667): p. 911-8.

[22] Kastrati, A., et al., *Analysis of 14 trials comparing sirolimus-eluting stents with bare-metal stents.* N Engl J Med, 2007. 356(10): p. 1030-9.

[23] Stone, G.W., et al., *Comparison of a polymer-based paclitaxel-eluting stent with a bare metal stent in patients with complex coronary artery disease: a randomized controlled trial.* JAMA, 2005. 294(10): p. 1215-23.

[24] Palmerini, T., et al., *Stent thrombosis with drug-eluting and bare-metal stents: evidence from a comprehensive network meta-analysis.* Lancet, 2012. 379(9824): p. 1393-402.

[25] Frutkin, A.D., et al., *Drug-eluting stents and the use of percutaneous coronary intervention among patients with class I indications for coronary artery bypass surgery undergoing index revascularization: analysis from the NCDR (National Cardiovascular Data Registry).* JACC Cardiovasc Interv, 2009. 2(7): p. 614-21.

[26] Wijns, W., et al., *Guidelines on myocardial revascularization.* Eur Heart J, 2010. 31(20): p. 2501-55.

[27] Yusuf, S., et al., *Effect of coronary artery bypass graft surgery on survival: overview of 10-year results from randomised trials by the Coronary Artery Bypass Graft Surgery Trialists Collaboration.* Lancet, 1994. 344(8922): p. 563-70.

[28] Dzavik, V., et al., *Long-term survival in 11,661 patients with multivessel coronary artery disease in the era of stenting: a report from the Alberta Provincial Project for Outcome Assessment in Coronary Heart Disease (APPROACH) Investigators.* Am Heart J, 2001. 142(1): p. 119-26.

[29] Baigent, C., et al., *Aspirin in the primary and secondary prevention of vascular disease: collaborative meta-analysis of individual participant data from randomised trials.* Lancet, 2009. 373(9678): p. 1849-60.

[30] Yusuf, S., et al., *Effects of clopidogrel in addition to aspirin in patients with acute coronary syndromes without ST-segment elevation.* N Engl J Med, 2001. 345(7): p. 494-502.

[31] Wiviott, S.D., et al., *Prasugrel versus clopidogrel in patients with acute coronary syndromes.* N Engl J Med, 2007. 357(20): p. 2001-15.

[32] Wallentin, L., et al., *Ticagrelor versus clopidogrel in patients with acute coronary syndromes.* N Engl J Med, 2009. 361(11): p. 1045-57.

[33] Packer, M., et al., *The effect of carvedilol on morbidity and mortality in patients with chronic heart failure. U.S. Carvedilol Heart Failure Study Group.* N Engl J Med, 1996. 334(21): p. 1349-55.

[34] *MRC/BHF Heart Protection Study of cholesterol lowering with simvastatin in 20,536 high-risk individuals: a randomised placebo-controlled trial.* Lancet, 2002. 360(9326): p. 7-22.

[35] LaRosa, J.C., et al., *Intensive lipid lowering with atorvastatin in patients with stable coronary disease.* N Engl J Med, 2005. 352(14): p. 1425-35.

[36] Yusuf, S., et al., *Effects of an angiotensin-converting-enzyme inhibitor, ramipril, on cardiovascular events in high-risk patients. The Heart Outcomes Prevention Evaluation Study Investigators.* N Engl J Med, 2000. 342(3): p. 145-53.

[37] Liu, M.W., G.S. Roubin, and S.B. King, 3rd, *Restenosis after coronary angioplasty. Potential biologic determinants and role of intimal hyperplasia.* Circulation, 1989. 79(6): p. 1374-87.

[38] Farb, A., et al., *Pathology of acute and chronic coronary stenting in humans.* Circulation, 1999. 99(1): p. 44-52.

[39] Colombo, A., et al., *Randomized study to assess the effectiveness of slow- and moderate-release polymer-based paclitaxel-eluting stents for coronary artery lesions.* Circulation, 2003. 108(7): p. 788-94.

[40] Morice, M.C., et al., *A randomized comparison of a sirolimus-eluting stent with a standard stent for coronary revascularization.* N Engl J Med, 2002. 346(23): p. 1773-80.

[41] Moses, J.W., et al., *Sirolimus-eluting stents versus standard stents in patients with stenosis in a native coronary artery.* N Engl J Med, 2003. 349(14): p. 1315-23.

[42] Stone, G.W., et al., *Safety and efficacy of sirolimus- and paclitaxel-eluting coronary stents*. N Engl J Med, 2007. 356(10): p. 998-1008.

[43] Pfisterer, M., et al., *Late clinical events after clopidogrel discontinuation may limit the benefit of drug-eluting stents: an observational study of drug-eluting versus bare-metal stents*. J Am Coll Cardiol, 2006. 48(12): p. 2584-91.

[44] Sarno, G., et al., *Lower risk of stent thrombosis and restenosis with unrestricted use of 'new-generation' drug-eluting stents: a report from the nationwide Swedish Coronary Angiography and Angioplasty Registry (SCAAR)*. Eur Heart J, 2012. 33(5): p. 606-13.

[45] Hlatky, M.A., et al., *Coronary artery bypass surgery compared with percutaneous coronary interventions for multivessel disease: a collaborative analysis of individual patient data from ten randomised trials*. Lancet, 2009. 373(9670): p. 1190-7.

[46] Passamani, E., et al., *A randomized trial of coronary artery bypass surgery. Survival of patients with a low ejection fraction*. N Engl J Med, 1985. 312(26): p. 1665-71.

[47] Scott, S.M., et al., *VA Study of Unstable Angina. 10-year results show duration of surgical advantage for patients with impaired ejection fraction*. Circulation, 1994. 90(5 Pt 2): p. II120-3.

[48] Velazquez, E.J., et al., *Coronary-artery bypass surgery in patients with left ventricular dysfunction*. N Engl J Med, 2011. 364(17): p. 1607-16.

[49] Gersh, B.J., et al., *2011 ACCF/AHA Guideline for the Diagnosis and Treatment of Hypertrophic Cardiomyopathy: a report of the American College of Cardiology Foundation/American Heart Association Task Force on Practice Guidelines. Developed in collaboration with the American Association for Thoracic Surgery, American Society of Echocardiography, American Society of Nuclear Cardiology, Heart Failure Society of America, Heart Rhythm Society, Society for Cardiovascular Angiography and Interventions, and Society of Thoracic Surgeons*. J Am Coll Cardiol, 2011. 58(25): p. e212-60.

[50] *Comparison of coronary bypass surgery with angioplasty in patients with multivessel disease. The Bypass Angioplasty Revascularization Investigation (BARI) Investigators*. N Engl J Med, 1996. 335(4): p. 217-25.

[51] Serruys, P.W., et al., *Percutaneous coronary intervention versus coronary-artery bypass grafting for severe coronary artery disease*. N Engl J Med, 2009. 360(10): p. 961-72.

[52] Chaitman, B.R., et al., *The Bypass Angioplasty Revascularization Investigation 2 Diabetes randomized trial of different treatment strategies in type 2 diabetes mellitus with stable ischemic heart disease: impact of treatment strategy on cardiac mortality and myocardial infarction*. Circulation, 2009. 120(25): p. 2529-40.

[53] Farkouh, M.E., et al., *Strategies for Multivessel Revascularization in Patients with Diabetes*. N Engl J Med, 2012.

[54] Hachamovitch, R., et al., *Comparison of the short-term survival benefit associated with revascularization compared with medical therapy in patients with no prior coronary artery dis-*

ease undergoing stress myocardial perfusion single photon emission computed tomography. Circulation, 2003. 107(23): p. 2900-7.

[55] Sorajja, P., et al., *Improved survival in asymptomatic diabetic patients with high-risk SPECT imaging treated with coronary artery bypass grafting.* Circulation, 2005. 112(9 Suppl): p. I311-6.

[56] Boden, W.E., et al., *Optimal medical therapy with or without PCI for stable coronary disease.* N Engl J Med, 2007. 356(15): p. 1503-16.

[57] Sianos, G., et al., *The SYNTAX Score: an angiographic tool grading the complexity of coronary artery disease.* EuroIntervention, 2005. 1(2): p. 219-27.

[58] Tu, J.V., et al., *Determinants of variations in coronary revascularization practices.* CMAJ, 2011.

[59] Kappetein, A.P., et al., *Comparison of coronary bypass surgery with drug-eluting stenting for the treatment of left main and/or three-vessel disease: 3-year follow-up of the SYNTAX trial.* Eur Heart J, 2011. 32(17): p. 2125-34.

[60] Rodriguez, A.E., et al., *Five-year follow-up of the Argentine randomized trial of coronary angioplasty with stenting versus coronary bypass surgery in patients with multiple vessel disease (ERACI II).* J Am Coll Cardiol, 2005. 46(4): p. 582-8.

[61] Hueb, W., et al., *Ten-year follow-up survival of the Medicine, Angioplasty, or Surgery Study (MASS II): a randomized controlled clinical trial of 3 therapeutic strategies for multivessel coronary artery disease.* Circulation, 2010. 122(10): p. 949-57.

[62] Hsieh, V. and S.R. Mehta, *How Should We Treat Multi-Vessel Disease in STEMI Patients?* Curr Treat Options Cardiovasc Med, 2012.

[63] Vlaar, P.J., et al., *Culprit vessel only versus multivessel and staged percutaneous coronary intervention for multivessel disease in patients presenting with ST-segment elevation myocardial infarction: a pairwise and network meta-analysis.* J Am Coll Cardiol, 2011. 58(7): p. 692-703.

[64] Hochman, J.S., et al., *Early revascularization in acute myocardial infarction complicated by cardiogenic shock. SHOCK Investigators. Should We Emergently Revascularize Occluded Coronaries for Cardiogenic Shock.* N Engl J Med, 1999. 341(9): p. 625-34.

[65] Hochman, J.S., et al., *One-year survival following early revascularization for cardiogenic shock.* JAMA, 2001. 285(2): p. 190-2.

[66] Hochman, J.S., et al., *Early revascularization and long-term survival in cardiogenic shock complicating acute myocardial infarction.* JAMA, 2006. 295(21): p. 2511-5.

[67] Mehta, R.H., et al., *Percutaneous coronary intervention or coronary artery bypass surgery for cardiogenic shock and multivessel coronary artery disease?* Am Heart J, 2010. 159(1): p. 141-7.

[68] Patel, M.R., et al., *ACCF/SCAI/STS/AATS/AHA/ASNC/HFSA/SCCT 2012 Appropriate use criteria for coronary revascularization focused update: a report of the American College of Cardiology Foundation Appropriate Use Criteria Task Force, Society for Cardiovascular Angiography and Interventions, Society of Thoracic Surgeons, American Association for Thoracic Surgery, American Heart Association, American Society of Nuclear Cardiology, and the Society of Cardiovascular Computed Tomography*. J Am Coll Cardiol, 2012. 59(9): p. 857-81.

[69] Baim, D.S., *Anatomy, Angiograpic Views and Quantitation of Stenosis*. Cardiac Catheterization, Angiography and Intervention, ed. D.S. Baim. Vol. Seventh Edition. 2006: Lippincott Williams and Wilkins.

[70] Uren, N.G., et al., *Relation between myocardial blood flow and the severity of coronary-artery stenosis*. N Engl J Med, 1994. 330(25): p. 1782-8.

[71] Pijls, N.H., et al., *Experimental basis of determining maximum coronary, myocardial, and collateral blood flow by pressure measurements for assessing functional stenosis severity before and after percutaneous transluminal coronary angioplasty*. Circulation, 1993. 87(4): p. 1354-67.

[72] Pijls, N.H. and J.W. Sels, *Functional measurement of coronary stenosis*. J Am Coll Cardiol, 2012. 59(12): p. 1045-57.

[73] Tonino, P.A., et al., *Fractional flow reserve versus angiography for guiding percutaneous coronary intervention*. N Engl J Med, 2009. 360(3): p. 213-24.

[74] Pijls, N.H., et al., *Fractional flow reserve versus angiography for guiding percutaneous coronary intervention in patients with multivessel coronary artery disease: 2-year follow-up of the FAME (Fractional Flow Reserve Versus Angiography for Multivessel Evaluation) study*. J Am Coll Cardiol, 2010. 56(3): p. 177-84.

[75] Ko, D.T., et al., *Temporal trends in the use of percutaneous coronary intervention and coronary artery bypass surgery in New York State and Ontario*. Circulation, 2010. 121(24): p. 2635-44.

[76] Hassan, A., et al., *Increasing rates of angioplasty versus bypass surgery in Canada, 1994-2005*. Am Heart J, 2010. 160(5): p. 958-65.

[77] McMurtry, M.S., et al., *Recent Temporal Trends and Geographic Distribution of Cardiac Procedures in Alberta*. Can J Cardiol, 2012.

[78] Riley, R.F., et al., *Trends in coronary revascularization in the United States from 2001 to 2009: recent declines in percutaneous coronary intervention volumes*. Circ Cardiovasc Qual Outcomes, 2011. 4(2): p. 193-7.

[79] Mercuri, M., et al., *An even smaller area variation: Differing practice patterns among interventional cardiologists within a single high volume tertiary cardiac centre*. Health Policy, 2012. 104(2): p. 179-85.

[80] Brown, R., et al., *Variation in Interventional Cardiac Care in Michigan.* Center for Healthcare research and Transformation, Ann Arbor, MI., 2012.

[81] Tu, J.V., et al., *Determinants of variations in coronary revascularization practices.* CMAJ, 2012. 184(2): p. 179-86.

[82] Schwalm, J., Lai, TF, Al-Haarbi, A, Karl D, Guo H, Kingsbury K, Tu JV, Natarajan MK, *Comparison of abstracted chart review and core-lab angiogram review on coronary angiography interpretation - an analysis from the variation in revascularization practice in ontario angiographic sub-study.* Canadian Cardiovascular Congress, 2010. Abstract presentation.

Chapter 3

Artery Bypass Versus PCI Using New Generation DES

Mohammed Balghith

Additional information is available at the end of the chapter

1. Introduction

Stents have substantially improved the safety and efficacy of percutaneous revascularization of atherosclerotic coronary arteries. The attendant risk of emergency referral for Coronary artery bypass graft surgery (CABG) and the need for subsequent revascularization procedures have been reduced by more than 50% since the use of new generation stents i.e drug eluted stents (DES) starting 2002. Comparisons of Percatouneous coronary intervention (PCI) and CABG have been made in 7 randomized trials designed to identify the most effective alternative for selected patients with multivessel CAD of whom both methods were deemed feasible. [1,2]. The individual results of these trials and a meta-analysis of their combined results have consistently shown equivalent survival rates with use of the 2 strategies over approximately 5 years of follow-up.

2. Coronary artery bypass graft surgery

A coronary artery bypass surgery is a surgical procedure performed to relieve angina and reduce the risk of death from coronary artery disease. Arteries or veins from elsewhere in the patient's body are grafted to the coronary arteries to bypass atherosclerotic narrowings and improve the blood supply to the coronary circulation supplying the myocardium (heart muscle). Example, Left internal mammary artery (LIMA) graft to LAD and SVG to OM and RCA (figure 1). The operation is usually performed with the heart stopped, requiring the usage of cardiopulmonary bypass; other methods are available to achieve CABG on a beating heart, so-called "off-pump" surgery. [3].

3. Advantages of CABG

Over the last 4 decades, surgical coronary artery revascularization techniques and technology have advanced significantly. As a result, despite an increasingly older and sicker patient population, CABG outcomes continue to improve. For example, the predicted mortality of CABG patients has increased steadily over the past decade, yet observed operative mortality rates have decreased, [4]. This is partly because advances in preoperative evaluation, including more precise coronary artery and myocardial imaging and diagnostic techniques, have allowed more appropriate patient selection and surgical planning. In addition, preoperative, intraoperative, and postoperative monitoring and therapeutic interventions have made CABG safer, even for critically ill and high-risk patients. Improvements in cardiopulmonary perfusion and careful myocardial protection, as well as the use of off-pump and on-pump beating-heart techniques in selected patients, have also decreased perioperative morbidity and mortality rates. [5,6].

Use of the bilateral IMAs offers the possibility of constructing various configurations, making total arterial myocardial revascularisation possible with a minimum number of arterial conduits. Use of the skeletonised RIMA through the transverse sinus and eventually retrocavally can reach most branches of the circumflex system and is associated with an excellent patency rate. Patients who received bilateral IMA grafts for left coronary system revascularisation had improved early and late outcomes and decreased risk of death, reoperation, and angioplasty. [7].

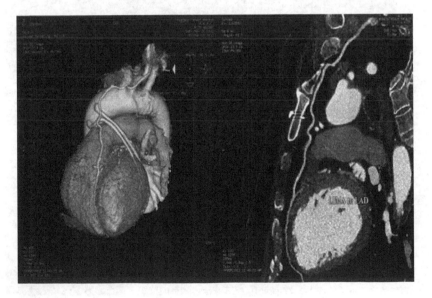

Figure 1. CT coronary angiogram, showing a CABG done 5 years ago with LIMA to LAD artery and SVG to OM and RCA.

4. Percutaneous coronary intervention using drug eluted stents

Percutaneous coronary intervention (PCI) involves dilatation of an obstructed or narrowed coronary artery, using a balloon catheter to dilate the artery from within. After balloon dilatation, a stainless steel stent is usually placed in the coronary artery. Antiplatelet agents like aspirin or clopidogrel are mandatory to be used after stenting. Stents may be either bare metal (BMS) or drug-eluting stents (DES). Indications for PCI might be elective or emergency according to the clinical presentations of the patients. Primary PCI in the setting of ST segment elevation myocardial infarction (STEMI): When the catheterization lab including the team and facility is available, angioplasty with stenting is the optimal method of reperfusion for STEMI. The target "door to balloon time" is 90 minutes, [8]. Rescue PCI is considered as a treatment in patients with thrombolysis - if there is failure to reperfuse, further ischaemia with persistant chest pain, or continuous ST elevation. PCI is considered also as an early invasive strategy in Acute coronary syndrome, Non-ST elevation myocardial infarction (NSTEMI) and unstable angina: [9]., or conservative strategy for patients who are at medium-to-high risk of subsequent cardiac events. Elective PCI for patient with Stable angina or positive stress test: with single or double vessel disease, where optimal medical therapy fails to control symptoms. Patients with triple vessel disease, who are unsuitable for CABG, [10].

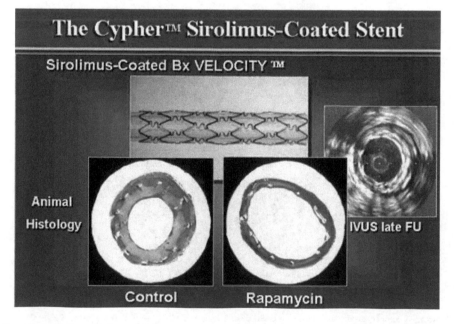

Figure 2. Cypher Stent- Siroliums eluted stent

A drug-eluting stent presents or releases single or multiple bioactive agents into the blood stream. The drug can deposit in and/or affect blood vessels, cells, plaque, or tissues either adjacent to the stent or at a distance. The drug can be embedded and released from within ("matrix-type") or surrounded by and released through ("reservoir-type") polymer materials that coat ("strut-adherent") or span ("strut-spanning") the struts of the stents. These agents prevent in-stent restenosis by reducing the intimal hyperplasia, [11].

The advantages and a lower cost compared to CABG makes DES an attractive option to treat coronary artery disease. Currently, five DESs are available in the USA: the CYPHER sirolimus-eluting stent from Cordis (approved by FDA on 24 April 2003), Figure 2, 3. The TAXUS Express and Liberté paclitaxel-eluting stents from Boston Scientific (approved by FDA on 4 March 2004 and 10 October 2008, respectively) (TAXUS Express is referred to as TAXUS) Figure 4, the ENDEAVOR zotarolimus-eluting stent from Medtronic (approved by FDA on 1 February 2008), and the XIENCE V Figure 5, everolimus-eluting stent from Abbott Vascular (approved by FDA on 2 July 2008). [12].

Figure 3. Complex case with LM disease treated by 2 Cypher stents

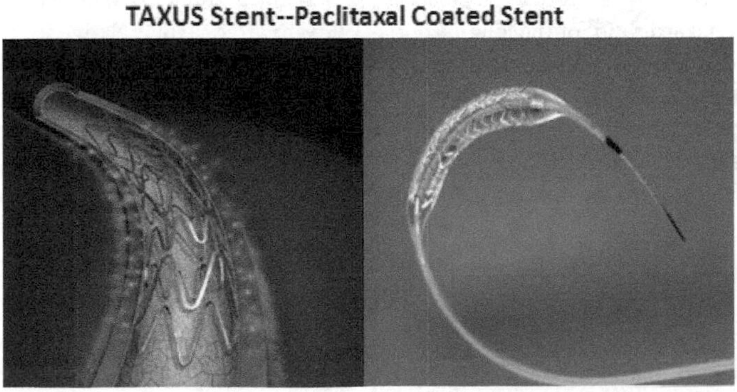

TAXUS Stent--Paclitaxal Coated Stent

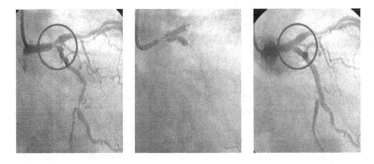

Figure 4. Taxus stent-Paclitaxal eluted stent

RCA 99% stenosis treated by Xience stent

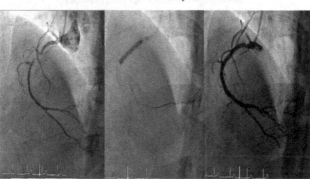

Figure 5. Significan disease of proximal RCA treated by Xience stent

5. Outcomes of coronary-artery bypass grafting versus bare metal stent implantation

The New York's cardiac registries were one of the largest studies which identify 37,212 patients with multivessel disease who underwent CABG and 22,102 patients with multivessel disease who underwent PCI using BMS from January 1, 1997, to December 31, 2000. They determined the rates of death and subsequent revascularization within three years after the procedure in various groups of patients according to the number of diseased vessels and presence or absence of involvement of the left anterior descending coronary artery LAD.

Risk-adjusted survival rates were significantly higher among patients who underwent CABG than among those who received a stent in all of the anatomical subgroups studied. For example, the adjusted hazard ratio for the long-term risk of death after CABG relative to stent implantation was 0.64 (95 percent confidence interval, 0.56 to 0.74) for patients with three-vessel disease with involvement of the proximal LAD and 0.76 (95 percent confidence interval, 0.60 to 0.96) for patients with two-vessel disease with involvement of the non-proximal LAD. Also, the three-year rates of revascularization were considerably higher in the stenting group than in the CABG group (7.8 percent vs. 0.3 percent for subsequent CABG and 27.3 percent vs. 4.6 percent for subsequent PCI), [13].

Texas Heart Institute Cardiovascular Research Database retrospectively identified patients who had undergone their 1st revascularization procedure with coronary artery bypass surgery (CABG; n=2,826) or coronary stenting (n=2,793) between January 1995 and December 1999. They have found that in-hospital mortality was significantly greater in patients undergoing CABG than in those undergoing stenting (3.6% vs 0.75%; adjusted OR 8.4; P <0.0001). At a mean 2.5-year follow-up, risk-adjusted survival was equivalent (CABG 91%, stenting 95%;

adjusted OR 1.26; P = 0.06). When subgroups matched for severity of disease were compared, no differences in risk-adjusted survival were seen, [14].

6. Drug-eluting stents vs coronary artery bypass surgery for the treatment of multivessel coronary disease

A Chinese study identified 3720 consecutive patients with multivessel disease who underwent isolated CABG surgery or received drug-eluting stents between April 1, 2004, and December 31, 2005, which compared safety (total mortality, myocardial infarction, and stroke) and efficacy (target-vessel revascularization) during a 3-year follow-up. These outcomes were compared after adjustment for the differences in baseline risk factors. Patients who underwent CABG (n=1886) were older and had more comorbidities than patients who received drug-eluting stents (n=1834). Patients receiving drug-eluting stents had considerably higher 3-year rates of target-vessel revascularization. Drug-eluting stents were also associated with higher rates of death (adjusted hazard ratio, 1.62; 95% confidence interval, 1.07 to 2.47) and myocardial infarction (adjusted hazard ratio, 1.65; 95% confidence interval, 1.15 to 2.44). The risk adjusted rate of stroke was similar in the 2 groups (hazard ratio, 0.92; 95% confidence interval, 0.69 to 1.51). [15]

In a Korean study, a 5-year clinical follow-up of 395 patients with unprotected LMCA disease who underwent PCI with drug-eluting stents (DES) (n = 176) or CABG (n = 219) was preformed from January 2003 to May 2004. In the 5-year follow up, cohort of DES and concurrent CABG, there had not been a significant difference in the adjusted risk of death (HR: 0.83; 95% CI: 0.34 to 2.07; p = 0.70) or the risk of the composite outcome (HR: 0.91; 95% CI: 0.45 to 1.83; p = 0.79). The rates of TVR were also higher in the DES group than the CABG group (HR: 6.22; 95% CI: 2.26 to 17.14; p < 0.001), [16].

In an Italian study, 249 patients: 107 of whom were treated with PCI along with DES implantation and 142 treated with CABG. At 5-year clinical follow-up, no difference was found between PCI and CABG in the occurrence of cardiac death (adjusted odds ratio [OR]: 0.502; 95% confidence interval [CI]: 0.162 to 1.461; p = 0.24). The PCI group showed a trend toward a lower occurrence of the composite end point of cardiac death and MI (adjusted OR: 0.408; 95% CI: 0.146 to 1.061; p = 0.06). Percutaneous coronary intervention was associated with a lower rate of the composite end point of death, MI, and/or stroke (OR: 0.399; 95% CI: 0.151 to 0.989; p = 0.04). Indeed, CABG was correlated with lower target vessel revascularization (adjusted OR: 4.411; 95% CI: 1.825 to 11.371; p = 0.0004). No difference was detected in the occurrence of major adverse cardiac and cerebrovascular events (adjusted OR: 1.578; 95% CI: 0.825 to 3.054; p = 0.18) [17].

In a Meta-analysis of clinical studies comparing CABG with DES in patients with unprotected left main coronary artery narrowing, the analysis included 2,905 patients from 8 clinical studies (2 randomized trials and 6 nonrandomized studies). At 1-year follow-up, there was no significant difference between the CABG and DES groups in the risk for death (odds ratio [OR] 1.12, 95% confidence interval [CI] 0.80 to 1.56) or the composite end point of death, myocardial infarction, or stroke (OR 1.25, 95% CI 0.86 to 1.82). The risk for target vessel revascularization was significantly lower in the CABG group compared to the PCI group (OR 0.44, 95% CI 0.32 to 0.59). In conclusion, PCI with DES is safe and could represent a good alternative to CABG for selected cases in patients with ULMCA disease, [18].

In the SYNTAX trial, 1,800 patients with three-vessel and/or LM disease were randomized to either CABG or PCI; of these, 271 LM patients were prospectively assigned to receive a 15-month angiogram. The primary endpoint for the CABG arm was the ratio of ≥50% to <100% obstructed/occluded grafts bypassing LM lesions to the number placed. The primary endpoint for the PCI arm was the proportion of patients with ≤50% diameter stenosis ('patent' stents) of treated LM lesions. Per protocol, no formal comparison between CABG and PCI arms was intended based on the differing primary endpoints. Available 15-month angiograms were analyzed for 114 CABG and 149 PCI patients. At 15 months, 9.9% (26/263) of CABG grafts were 100% occluded and an additional 5.7% (15/263) were ≥50% to <100% occluded. Overall, 27.2% (31/114) of patients had ≥1 obstructed/occluded graft. The 15-month CABG MACCE rate was 8.8% (10/114) and MACCE at 15 months was not significantly associated with graft obstruction/occlusion (p=0.85). In the PCI arm, 92.4% (134/145) of patients had ≤50% diameter LM stenosis at 15 months (89.7% [87/97] distal LM lesions and 97.9% [47/48] non-distal LM lesions). The 15-month PCI MACCE rate was 12.8% (20/156) and this was significantly associated with lack of stent patency at 15 months (p<0.001), mainly due to repeated revascularization. [19].

The results of the SYNTAX trial confirm that at 3 years CABG remains the treatment of choice for most patients with three-vessel and LMS disease and especially in those with the most severe disease. SYNTAX will have a profound effect on practice recommendations for the foreseeable future and has already had a major effect on the new European Society for Cardiology/European Association for Cardiothoracic Surgery guidelines for myocardial revascularization, [20].

At four years follow-up of SYNTAX trial which presented at TCT in 2011, there was no difference in MACCE between CABG and PCI in those with a SYNTAX score of 0 to 22, (26.1% vs 28.6%; p=0.57). This is good, and would legitimize the use of PCI in this kind of patient". But for those with an intermediate SYNTAX score of 23 to 32, "You see immediately a highly significant difference" in MACCE rate (21.5% for CABG vs 32% for PCI; p=0.006). For those with a high SYNTAX score (≥33), "mortality is double in the PCI group compared with CABG (16.1% vs 8.4%; p=0.04) in addition to MI is two to three times higher with PCI than with CABG (9.3% vs 3.9%; p=0.01).

In this highest-risk group, even the end point of death/stroke/MI becomes significantly higher with PCI, (22.7% vs 14.6%; p=0.01), and MACCE were much higher (40.1% vs 23.6%; p<0.001), driven in large part by a 17% higher rate of revascularization in this high-risk group at four years. Figures 6& 7

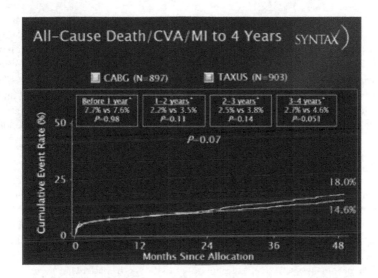

Figure 6. years follow up in Syntax study, demonstrate all cause death/CVA/MI up to 4 years

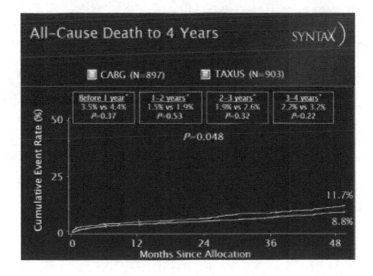

Figure 7. years follow up in Syntax study, demonstrate all cause death up to 4 years

7. Revascularization for patients with diabetes mellitus and multivessel CAD

In the BARI 2D trial, the selected revascularization strategy, CABG or PCI, was based on physician discretion, declared independent of randomization to either immediate or deferred revascularization if clinically warranted. They analyzed factors favoring selection of CABG versus PCI in 1,593 diabetic patients with multivessel CAD enrolled between 2001 and 2005. The majority of diabetic patients with multivessel disease were selected for PCI rather than CABG. Preference for CABG over PCI was largely based on angiographic features related to the extent, location, and nature of CAD, as well as geographic, demographic, and clinical factors. [21]

However, with each intervention the benefit is less and the risks and complications are greater than in patients without diabetes. Revascularization for treatment of ST elevation myocardial infarction increases survival. Both interventions relieve symptoms, but neither improves survival except in patients at high risk. In patients with clinically stable chronic coronary disease, survival after CABG or PCI is comparable with that in patients treated with optimal medical therapy alone. Accordingly, evaluation for revascularization can be deferred until signs and symptoms worsen except in patients at high risk. In patients at high risk survival after promptly implemented CABG is greater than that with optimal medical therapy, especially when the diabetes is being treated with insulin sensitizing agents. [22]

8. Quality of life after PCI with DES or CABG

Among patients with three-vessel or left main coronary artery disease who were suitable candidates for either PCI using DES or CABG, both strategies resulted in significant relief from angina and improvements in overall health status over the first year of follow-up. At both 6 and 12 months, there was a small but significant reduction in angina frequency with CABG as compared with PCI in the overall population. These symptomatic benefits of CABG were counterbalanced by the more rapid recovery and improved short-term health status achieved with PCI. [23]

9. Future study with the second generation des and other bioabsorbable stents

EXCEL is a 2600-patient study comparing patients with left main disease randomized to bypass surgery or PCI with the Xience stent and followed for at least three years. The primary end point is death, stroke, and MI; repeat revascularization is a secondary end point. EXCEL results awaited. Figure (8)

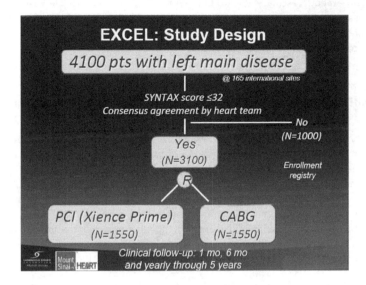

Figure 8. EXCEL study protocol comparing Xience stent with CABG

The BVS everolimus-eluting stent system

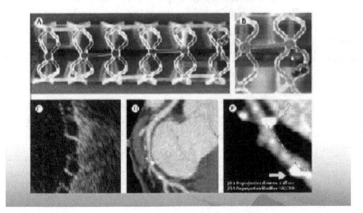

Figure 9. Absorb Stent- Bioabsorbale everolimus eluted stent

Stents composed of bioabsorbable/biodegradable materials represent an attractive alternative revascularization modality; the justification stems from the short-term need for vessel scaffolding and avoidance of the potential long-term complications of metallic stents. Compared with metallic stents, there are several potential advantages, including complete absorption of stent material, [24], Abbott Vascular ABSORB Everolimus Eluting Bioresorbable Vascular Scaffold System"These outcomes suggest that a temporary scaffold like ABSORB provides durable results over the long term and a permanent implant may not be necessary to effectively treat patients with coronary artery disease". ABSORB II trial is ongoing. Figure (9)

10. Combining the best of both worlds hybrid coronary revascularization

As PCI technology improves and techniques of LIMA-to-LAD grafting become less invasive, hybrid coronary revascularization is becoming a distinct possibility. For example, a minimally invasive, off-pump, direct LIMA-to-LAD anastomosis can be combined with DES placement in a focal mid-right-coronary-artery lesion in a patient with complex proximal LAD lesions. Hybrid coronary revascularization procedures are currently being performed, with promising early results. A few centers, now have hybrid operating rooms with cardiac surgical and coronary angiographic capabilities that make it possible to perform simultaneous hybrid coronary revascularizations. Staged hybrid revascularizations are performed in standard catheterization laboratories and operating rooms. [25,26].

11. Conclusion

Each strategy can have great outcomes in appropriately selected patients. Hard clinical outcomes (death/MI/CVA) are generally similar, need to weigh the risk of potential repetition of procedures with PCI using DES vs. the greater morbidity of CABG. The 3VD and LMCA Disease are high-risk coronary lesions and the least stable subtypes of "stable CAD" PCI and CABG have very similar rates of hard clinical endpoints. Greater rates of recurrent revascularization with PCI, especially in complex disease, Patient selection and patient preference will generally dictate the best and most appropriate care. The so-called SYNTAX score, evolved for the trial, offers a grading system, based on patient anatomy, to help surgeons and interventionalists make this decision. As PCI and CABG are refined further, surgeons and cardiologists will no doubt learn to use these improved interventional techniques and surgical procedures in a way that will optimize the treatment of each individual patient.

Author details

Mohammed Balghith

King Saud Bin Abdulaziz University for Heath Sceinces, KACC, National Guard , Riyadh, Saudi Arabia

References

[1] Rodriguez A, Boullon F, Perez-Balino N, Paviotti C, Liprandi MI, Palacios IF. Argentine randomized trial of percutaneous transluminal coronary angioplasty versus coronary artery bypass surgery in multivessel disease (ERACI): in-hospital results and 1-year follow-up. ERACI Group. J Am Coll Cardiol 1993;22:1060–7.

[2] Hamm CW, Reimers J, Ischinger T, Rupprecht HJ, Berger J, Bleifeld W. A randomized study of coronary angioplasty compared with bypass surgery in patients with symptomatic multivessel coronary disease. German Angioplasty Bypass Surgery Investigation (GABI). N Engl J Med 1994;331: 1037–43

[3] Kolessov et al, "Mammary artery-coronary artery anastomosis as method of treatment for angina pectoris". J Thorac Cardiovasc Surg VI (October 1967). 54 (4): 535–44

[4] Ferguson TB Jr, Hammill BG, Peterson ED, DeLong ER, Grover FL, STS National Database Committee. A decade of change: risk profiles and outcomes for isolated coronary artery bypass grafting procedures, 1990–1999: a report from the STS National Database Committee and the Duke Clinical Research Institute. Society of Thoracic Surgeons. Ann Thorac Surg 2002;73:480–9.

[5] Al-Ruzzeh S, Ambler G, Asimakopoulos G, Omar RZ, Hasan R, Fabri B, et al. Off-pump coronary artery bypass (OPCAB) surgery reduces risk-stratified morbidity and mortality: a United Kingdom multi-center comparative analysis of early clinical outcome. Circulation 2003;108 Suppl 1:II1–8.

[6] Puskas JD, Williams WH, Mahoney EM, Huber PR, Block PC, Duke PG, et al. Off-pump vs conventional coronary artery bypass grafting: early and 1-year graft patency, cost, and quality-of-life outcomes: a randomized trial. JAMA 2004;291:1841–9.

[7] M Bonacchi, Battaglia F, Prifti E, Leacche M, Nathan N S, Sani G, and Popoff G,Early and late outcome of skeletonised bilateral internal mammary arteries anastomosed to the left coronary system Heart. 2005 February; 91(2): 195–202. Ratcliffe A T, C Pepper. Thrombolysis or primary angioplasty? Reperfusion therapy for myocardial infarction in the UK, Postgrad Med J2008;84:73-77

[8] Ratcliffe A T , C Pepper . Thrombolysis or primary angioplasty? Reperfusion therapy for myocardial infarction in the UK, Postgrad Med J2008;84:73-77

[9] McCullough PA, Gibson CM, Dibattiste PM, et al. Timing of angiography and revascularization in acute coronary syndromes: an analysis of the TACTICS-TIMI-18 trial. J Interv Cardiol 2004;17:81-6

[10] Levine GN, Bates ER, Blankenship JC, et al. 2011 ACCF/AHA/SCAI guideline for percutaneous coronary intervention: A report of the American College of Cardiology Foundation/American Heart Association Task Force on Practice Guidelines and the

Society for Cardiovascular Angiography and Interventions. J Am Coll Cardiol 2011;08.007

[11] Robert S. Schwartz, MD; Elazer R. Edelman, MD, PhD; Andrew Carter, DO; Nicolas Chronos, MD; Campbell Rogers, MD; Keith A. Robinson, PhD; Ron Waksman, MD; Judah Weinberger, MD; Robert L. Wilensky, MD; Donald N. Jensen, DVM; Bram D. Zuckerman, MD; Renu VirmaniDrug-Eluting Stents in Preclinical Studies, Recommended Evaluation From a Consensus Group, Circulation. 2002; 106: 1867-1873

[12] Doostzadeh J, Clark LN, Bezenek S, Pierson W, Sood PR, Sudhir K. Recent progress in percutaneous coronary intervention: evolution of the drug-eluting stents, focus on the XIENCE V drug-eluting stent. Coron Artery Dis. 2010 Jan;21(1):46-56.

[13] Hannan EL, Racz MJ, Walford G, Jones RH, Ryan TJ, Bennett E, Culliford AT, Isom OW, Gold JP, Rose EA, N Engl J Med. Long-term outcomes of coronary-artery bypass grafting versus stent implantation. 2005 May 26;352(21):2174-83.

[14] Rollo P. Villareal, MD, Vei-Vei Lee, MS, MacArthur A. Elayda, MD, PhD, and James M. Wilson, MD Coronary Artery Bypass Surgery versus Coronary Stenting, Risk-Adjusted Survival Rates in 5,619 Patients. Tex Heart Inst J. 2002; 29(1): 3–9

[15] Li Y, Zheng Z, Xu B, Zhang S, Li W, Gao R, Hu S.Comparison of drug-eluting stents and coronary artery bypass surgery for the treatment of multivessel coronary disease: three-year follow-up results from a single institution. Circulation. 2009 Apr 21;119(15):2040-50

[16] Park DW, Kim YH, Yun SC, Lee JY, Kim WJ, Kang SJ, Lee SW, Lee CW, Kim JJ, Choo SJ, Chung CH, Lee JW, Park SW, Park SJ. Long-term outcomes after stenting versus coronary artery bypass grafting for unprotected left main coronary artery disease: 10-year results of bare-metal stents and 5-year results of drug-eluting stents from the ASAN-MAIN (ASAN Medical Center-Left MAIN Revascularization) Registry. J Am Coll Cardiol. 2010 Oct 19;56(17):1366-75.

[17] Chieffo A, Magni V, Latib A, Maisano F, Ielasi A, Montorfano M, Carlino M, Godino C, Ferraro M, Calori G, Alfieri O, Colombo A. 5-year outcomes following percutaneous coronary intervention with drug-eluting stent implantation versus coronary artery bypass graft for unprotected left main coronary artery lesions the Milan experience. JACC Cardiovasc Interv. 2010 Jun;3(6):595-601.

[18] Lee MS, Yang T, Dhoot J, Liao H. Meta-analysis of clinical studies comparing coronary artery bypass grafting with percutaneous coronary intervention and drug-eluting stents in patients with unprotected left main coronary artery narrowings. Am J Cardiol. 2010 Apr 15;105(8).

[19] Morice MC, Feldman TE, Mack MJ, Ståhle E, Holmes DR, Colombo A, Morel MA, van den Brand M, Serruys PW, Mohr F, Carrié D, Fournial G, James S, Leadley K, Dawkins KD, Kappetein AP. Angiographic outcomes following stenting or coronary artery bypass surgery of the left main coronary artery: fifteen-month outcomes from

the synergy between PCI with TAXUS express and cardiac surgery left main angiographic substudy (SYNTAX-LE MANS). EuroIntervention. 2011 Oct 30;7(6):670-9.

[20] Taggart DP. Lessons learned from the SYNTAX trial for multivessel and left main stem coronary artery disease. Curr Opin Cardiol. 2011 Nov;26(6):502-7.

[21] Kim LJ, King SB 3rd, Kent K, Brooks MM et al; BARI 2D (Bypass Angioplasty Revascularization Investigation Type 2 Diabetes) Study Group.Factors related to the selection of surgical versus percutaneous revascularization in diabetic patients with multivessel coronary artery disease in the BARI 2D (Bypass Angioplasty Revascularization Investigation in Type 2 Diabetes) trial. JACC Cardiovasc Interv. 2009 May; 2(5):384-92.

[22] Sobel BE.Coronary revascularization in patients with type 2 diabetes and results of the BARI 2D trial. Coron Artery Dis. 2010 May;21(3):189-98.

[23] David J. Cohen, M.D., Ben Van Hout, Ph.D., Patrick W. Serruys, M.D., Ph.D., for the Synergy between PCI with Taxus and Cardiac Surgery (SYNTAX) Investigators, Quality of Life after PCI with Drug-Eluting Stents or Coronary-Artery Bypass Surgery. N Engl J Med 2011; 364:1016-1026March 17, 2011

[24] Waksman R, Erbel R, Di Mario C, et al; PROGRESS-AMS (Clinical Performance Angiographic Results of Coronary Stenting with Absorbable Metal Stents) Investigators. Early- and long-term intravascular ultrasound and angiographic findings after bioabsorbable magnesium stent implantation in human coronary arteries. JACC Cardiovasc Intervent. 2009;2:312-320

[25] de Canniere D, Jansens JL, Goldschmidt-Clermont P, Barvais L, Decroly P, Stoupel E. Combination of minimally invasive coronary bypass and percutaneous transluminal coronary angioplasty in the treatment of double-vessel coronary disease: two-year follow-up of a new hybrid procedure compared with "on-pump" double bypass grafting. Am Heart J 2001;142:563-70.

[26] Lee MS, Wilentz JR, Makkar RR, Singh V, Nero T, Swistel D, et al. Hybrid revascularization using percutaneous coronary intervention and robotically assisted minimally invasive direct coronary artery bypass surgery. J Invasive Cardiol 2004;16:419-25.

Peripheral and Cerebral Vascular Disease Intervention

Chapter 4

Infected Aneurysm and Inflammatory Aorta: Diagnosis and Management

Takao Kato

Additional information is available at the end of the chapter

1. Introduction

Due to the increase of aged patients with atherosclerosis, more attention should be paid to the endothelial damage of great vessels. The damaged endothelium is more susceptible to bacterial infections. The reports or papers of infected aneurysms (mycotic aneurysms) are increasing in Pubmed search (Figure 1), which is consistent with personal experience in daily practice. The reasons for the increase were due to several causes: 1) the increase of aged patients with more risk of atherosclerosis than before, 2) an improvement of CT imaging and MR imaging, 3) more awareness of the disease. We focused the diagnosis and managements of infected aneurysms, and the diseases needed to differentiate from infected aneurysms, such as collagen vascular diseases and periaortitis.

1.1. Diagnosis of infected aneurysms

Risk factors for infected aneurysm include: 1) Endothelial damage caused by atherosclerosis including pre-existing aneurysm [1], 2) Antecedent infection including bacteremia, 3) Arterial injury including iatrogenic mechanisms, such as percutaneous coronary intervention [2]. When the intima is diseased, bacteria can pass through it into deep layers of the aorta and can establish infection. Infective endocarditis (IE) remains to be main cause of infected aneurysm [3], because the risk factors of IE are very similar to those of infected aneurysms, and bacteremia and septic emboli from heart are often common features of IE.

Staphylococcus species (spp) and Salmonella spp are two major bacteria causing infected aneurysm, 28 to 71 percent and 15 to 24 percent of causes, respectively [4,5]. Streptococcus pneumoniae may be the third major, re-emerging, cause of infected aneurysms [6]. The pathology of the diseased site includes acute or chronic inflammation with bacterial infection, abscesses, and necrosis. The suprarenal abdominal aorta is most commonly involved site.

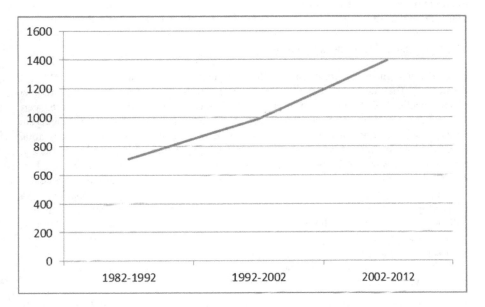

Figure 1. Results of Pubmed search using mycotic aneurysm or infected aneurysm.

Symptoms of an infected aneurysm vary according the lesion diseased. For example, abdominal pain and diarrhea is observed if abdominal aorta is involved, painful pulsatile mass if superficial artery is involved, and chest pain if thoracic aorta is involved. An infected aneurysm involving deep arteries or aorta may cause only fever. It might be followed as fever of unknown origin, and could be diagnosed as an infected aneurysm only after CT imaging is acquired. If the patients were with bacteremia or a persistent high fever and their etiology was not determined, the contrast-enhanced CT imaging would be the choice for searching the diseased lesion, and an asymptomatic infected aneurysm would be one of differential diagnoses.

The next step of diagnosing an infected aneurysm is based on blood cultures and imaging. In all suspicious patients, blood cultures should be examined. About 50-85% of patients may be positive [5,7]. If negative, however, the infected aneurysm cannot be ruled out. Contrast-enhanced CT imaging identified the infected aneurysm. Findings on CT angiography of an infected aneurysm include a disruption of aortic wall calcification, soft tissue inflammation or mass around a vessel, and periaortic fluid or air collection [8,9]. These findings can differentiate from other inflammatory aortic disease. The wall of inflammatory aorta is thickened and periaortic fibrosis sometimes observed in adhesion to surrounding organs. MR imaging is another strong tools. The T2-weighted images or mixed T1/T2-weighted STIR images are able to visualize the edematous lesion. The diffusion images can detect fluid collection, and gadolinium enhancement indicates the increase of inflammatory connective tissue.

In summary, the important things for the diagnosis of an infected aneurysm are the high suspicion of this disease and obtaining blood cultures and enhanced CT or MR imaging.

1.2. Management of infected aneurysms

Surgical replacement or debridement is the treatment of choice combined with antibiotic therapy [4]. The main aims of surgical procedures are removal of infected tissue and re-vascularization if distal perfusion is limited. Mortality rate without surgery was 85 percent with infected thoracic aneurysm and 96 percent with infected aortic aneurysm [10,11]. Figure 2 shows a gradually enlarged infective aneurysm treated on medication alone despite the control of bacteremia [12]. Among patients who underwent surgery, mortality rates were the highest for patients with infected arch aneurysms (50 %) compared with supra-renal aortic aneurysms (43%), distal descending thoracic aneurysms (33 %), proximal descending thoracic aneurysms (16 %), or infra-renal aortic aneurysms (4 %) [10,13]. Endovascular stenting is reported to be effective in some systematic reviews with low mortality [14,15]. Because the infected focus is not removed by endovascular stenting, the procedures may be palliative, and more persistent or recurrent infections are likely to occur compared to surgical procedures. However, endovascular procedures could be a secondary choice for patients who refuse surgery, those with a very high risk for surgery, and those with a ruptured infected aneurysm.

The initial choice of antibiotic therapy should be based on the culture and susceptibility results. Until the results become available, the combination treatment with vancomycin and a ceftriaxone, a fluoroquinolone, or piperacillin-tazobactam is preferable targeting gram-negative Salmonella and enteric bacteria. The optimal duration of antibiotic therapy is uncertain because of the lack of randomized clinical trials. In general, four to six weeks of parenteral antimicrobial therapy is performed for the treatment of infected aneurysm followed by principles of vascular graft infection or infective endocarditis of prosthesis valve. A longer duration of treatment or additional oral antibiotics may be warranted in the clinical course of persist elevation of C-reactive proteins or recurrence of fever when drug-related fever is excluded.

In summary, the surgical replacement in combination with antibiotics is the treatment of choice, and endovascular procedures may be palliative. The management is followed by principles of vascular graft infection or infective endocarditis of prosthesis valve.

2. Inflammation of aorta: "Aortits"

Large vessel vasculitits such as Takayasu's arteritis and giant cell arteritis, rheumatic and HLA-B27–associated spondyloarthropathies, Behçet's syndrome, and infections such as syphilis, tuberculosis may be the cause of inflammation of aorta, and we must differentiate these from infected aneurysms when blood culture is negative or infected focus remains unclear. Another disease which we must differentiate is IgG4-related diseases (chronic periaortits).

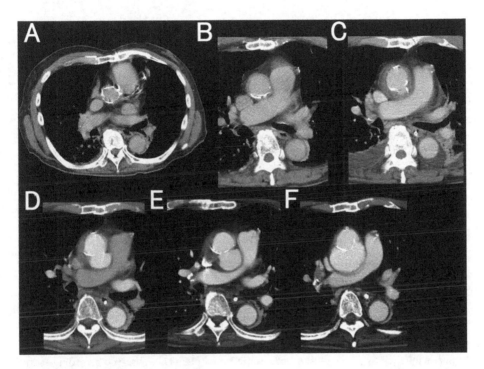

Figure 2. A case of medical treatment of an infected aneurysm. A 75-year-old man with familial hypercholesterolemia, cerebral infarction, and coronary bypass grafting presented with high fever and chest pain. Panel A and B showed a severely calcified ascending aorta. The repeated CE-CT on the 5th day revealed aneurysmal change with protrusion (Panel C), indicating an infected aneurysm. Due to a prohibitive risk of surgery, medical treatment was the choice of him and his family, but the infected aneurysm gradually enlarged despite the control of bacteremia with antibiotics (13th day: Panel D, 24th day: Panel E, and 58th day; Panel F), and he died 2 months after onset.

A detailed history and a careful physical examination are important for the diagnosis and assessment of the extent of vascular lesions. The mean age at onset of Takayasu's arteritis and giant cell arteritis was between 17 and 26 years of age and with 69 years, respectively, primarily in women (about 80 %) [16]. Systemic symptoms are common such as fatigue, weight loss, and low-grade fever are common in these disorders, along with local symptoms, for example, arthralgia, skin lesion (erythema nodosum), and abdominal pains. HLA-B27–associated spondyloarthropathies accompanies with ankylosing spondylitis, reactive arthritis, or inflammatory bowel disease with negative rheumatic factors. Skin and mucosa, ocular system, GI manifestations include abdominal pain, nausea, and diarrhea with or without blood, and/or musculoskeletal and neurological system are involved in Behçet's syndrome. Allergic features such as atopy, asthma, and modest peripheral eosinophilia, along with tumorous swelling in many organs and elevated serum IgG4 levels above the upper limit of normal(>135 mg/dL) are the characteristics of IgG-4 related diseases [17].

3. Takayasu's arteritis, giant cell arteritis

Takayasu's arteritis, also called pulseless disease, involves the ascending aorta and aortic arch, and carotid and subclavian arteries, causing dilations and obstruction at the stage of healing and recurrences. CT angiography revealed the diseased lesion, thickened arterial wall in acute phase and aneurysmal or stenotic lesion in chronic phase [18]. The ultrasonography and MR angiography are also useful. In acute phase, the high signal of T2-weighted and/or STIR MR images and the increased uptake of [18]Fluorodeoxy-glucose indicate the presence of active inflammation [19]. The mainstay of therapy for Takayasu's arteritis is glucocorticoids. Giant cell arteritis (GCA) is a chronic vasculitis of large and medium sized vessels. The following classification criteria were as follows: 1) Age older than 50 years at onset, 2) Localized headache de novo, 3) Tenderness or decreased pulse of the temporal artery, 4) Erythrocyte sedimentation rate (ESR) greater than 50 mm/h, 5) Biopsy-proven necrotizing arteritis with multinucleated giant cells [20].

4. IgG4-related diseases: Chronic periaortits

IgG4 -related disease is a newly recognized syndrome of unknown etiology characterized by fibroinflammatory condition, in which tumefactive lesions, a dense lymphoplasmacytic infiltrate rich in IgG4-positive plasma cells. Various symptoms are observed according to the lesions involved, although patients feel well at the time of diagnosis without fever. Seventy percent of patients have elevated serum IgG4 concentrations [17]. CT imaging features of arterial lesions are characterized by homogeneous wall thickening and enhancement in the late phases after contrast infusion accompanying the increase of connective tissue indicating sclerosing inflammation [21]. This indicates chronic periaortitis, which resembles the infected aneurysm with periaortic abscess (Figure 3). Therefore, the diseases should be differentiated from infected aneurysm by not only the imaging features but also clinical symptoms or negative blood cultures. Glucocorticoids typically the first line of therapy.

5. Conclusions

Due to the increase of aged patients with atherosclerosis, more attention should be paid to the endothelial damage of great vessels and an infected aneurysm should be properly diagnosed and carefully managed.

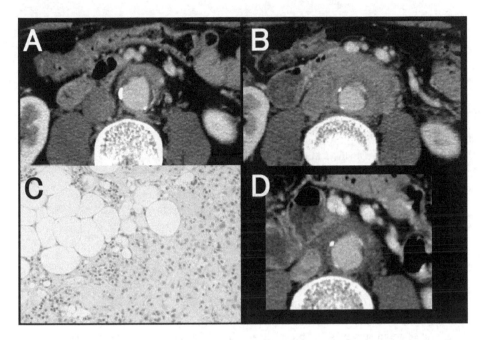

Figure 3. A case of chronic periaortitis with retroperitoneal fibrosis. A 75-year-old man presented with vague discomfort of lower abdomen. Panel A was at presentation. Two months later the symptoms remained unchanged with 8.5mg/dL of C-reactive protein but without fever. Repeated CT was performed (Panel B). Biopsy of the tissue revealed the infiltration of inflammatory cells and no bacteria (Panel C). Panel D was three weeks after the glucocorticoid therapy.

Disclosures

None.

Author details

Takao Kato*

Address all correspondence to: takao-kato@kitano-hp.or.jp

Cardiovascular Center, The Tazuke Kofukai Medical Research Institute, Kitano Hospital, Osaka, Japan

References

[1] Ernst CB, Campbell HC Jr, Daugherty ME, Sachatello CR, Griffen WO Jr. Incidence and significance of intra-operative bacterial cultures during abdominal aortic aneurysmectomy. Ann Surg 1977; 185: 626-33.

[2] Samore MH, Wessolossky MA, Lewis SM, Shubrooks SJ Jr, Karchmer AW. Frequency, risk factors, and outcome for bacteremia after percutaneous transluminal coronary angioplasty. Am J Cardiol 1997; 79:873-7.

[3] Johansen K, Devin J. Mycotic aortic aneurysms. A reappraisal. Arch Surg 1983; 118:583-8.

[4] Moneta GL, Taylor LM Jr, Yeager RA, Edwards JM, Nicoloff AD, McConnell DB, Porter JM. Surgical treatment of infected aortic aneurysm. Am J Surg 1998; 175:396-9.

[5] Johnson JR, Ledgerwood AM, Lucas CE. Mycotic aneurysm. New concepts in therapy. Arch Surg 1983; 118:577-82.

[6] Brouwer RE, van Bockel JH, van Dissel JT. Streptococcus pneumoniae, an emerging pathogen in mycotic aneurysms? Neth J Med 1998; 52:16-21.

[7] Maeda H, Umezawa H, Goshima M, Hattori T, Nakamura T, Umeda T, Shiono M. Primary infected abdominal aortic aneurysm: surgical procedures, early mortality rates, and a survey of the prevalence of infectious organisms over a 30-year period. Surg Today 2011; 41:346-51.

[8] Gomes MN, Choyke PL. Infected aortic aneurysms: CT diagnosis. J Cardiovasc Surg (Torino) 1992; 33:684-9.

[9] Lee WK, Mossop PJ, Little AF, Fitt GJ, Vrazas JI, Hoang JK, Hennessy OF. Infected (mycotic) aneurysms: spectrum of imaging appearances and management. Radiographics 2008; 28:1853-68.

[10] Weis-Müller BT, Rascanu C, Sagban A, Grabitz K, Godehardt E, Sandmann W. Single-center experience with open surgical treatment of 36 infected aneurysms of the thoracic, thoracoabdominal, and abdominal aorta. Ann Vasc Surg 2011; 25:1020-5.

[11] Taylor CF, Lennox AF. Treatment options for primary infected aorta. Ann Vasc Surg 2007; 21:225-7.

[12] Kato T, Kimura M, Inoko M, Nohara R. Infected aneurysm in an atherosclerotic lesion. Intern Med. 2012; 51:983.

[13] Lee CH, Hsieh HC, Ko PJ, Li HJ, Kao TC, Yu SY. In situ versus extra-anatomic reconstruction for primary infected infrarenal abdominal aortic aneurysms. J Vasc Surg 2011; 54:64-70.

[14] Kan CD, Lee HL, Yang YJ. Outcome after endovascular stent graft treatment for mycotic aortic aneurysm: a systematic review. J Vasc Surg 2007; 46:906-12.

[15] Kpodonu J, Williams JP, Ramaiah VG, Diethrich EB. Endovascular management of a descending thoracic mycotic aneurysm: mid-term follow-up. Eur J Cardiothorac Surg 2007; 32:178-9.

[16] Hunder GG, Arend WP, Bloch DA, Calabrese LH, Fauci AS, Fries JF, Leavitt RY, Lie JT, Lightfoot RW Jr, Masi AT, McShane DJ, Michel BA, Mills JA, Stevens MB, Wallace SL, Zvaifler NJ. The American College of Rheumatology 1990 criteria for the classification of vasculitis. Introduction. Arthritis Rheum 1990; 33:1065-7.

[17] Stone JH, Zen Y, Deshpande V. IgG4-related disease.N Engl J Med. 2012; 366:539-51.

[18] Yamada I, Nakagawa T, Himeno Y, Numano F, Shibuya H. Takayasu arteritis: evaluation of the thoracic aorta with CT angiography. Radiology 1998; 209:103-9.

[19] Kissin EY, Merkel PA. Diagnostic imaging in Takayasu arteritis. Curr Opin Rheumatol 2004; 16:31-7.

[20] Hunder GG, Bloch DA, Michel BA, Stevens MB, Arend WP, Calabrese LH, Edworthy SM, Fauci AS, Leavitt RY, Lie JT, et al. The American College of Rheumatology 1990 criteria for the classification of giant cell arteritis. Arthritis Rheum 1990; 33:1122-8.

[21] Inoue D, Zen Y, Abo H, Gabata T, Demachi H, Yoshikawa J, Miyayama S, Nakanuma Y, Matsui O. Immunoglobulin G4-related periaortitis and periarteritis: CT findings in 17 patients. Radiology 2011;251:625-33.

Chapter 5

Management of Carotid Artery Disease in the Setting of Coronary Artery Disease in Need of Coronary Artery Bypass Surgery

Aditya M. Sharma and Herbert D. Aronow

Additional information is available at the end of the chapter

1. Introduction

Coronary artery bypass graft surgery (CABG) is one of the most commonly performed major surgeries in the United States with over 397,000 CABG's performed in 2010.(Go, Mozaffarian et al. 2012) One of the most dreadful adverse sequelae of CABG is stroke which is also the 2nd most common major post-operative complication seen with CABG, occurring in 1 to 5% of patients.(Furlan, Sila et al. 1992; Brown, Kugelmass et al. 2008) Patients suffering from postoperative stroke have a very high incidence of in-hospital mortality.(Hogue, Murphy et al. 1999) Studies have shown that presence of extracranial carotid artery stenosis (ECAS) is a strong risk factor for post-operative morbidity and mortality due post-CABG strokes.(Brown, Kugelmass et al. 2008) In this book chapter, we will review the epidemiology of concomitant coronary and carotid artery disease, the association with post-operative stroke, recommendations for pre-operative ECAS screening and management options for patients in whom ECAS is identified.

Co-prevalence of carotid and coronary artery disease and its implications on perioperative and postoperative morbidity and mortality: Atherosclerosis is a systemic disease which is usually present in multiple vascular beds simultaneously.(Beique, Ali et al. 2006) In a recent study from the Cleveland Clinic involving 45,432 patient's, presence of carotid artery disease was confirmed as a significant risk factor for perioperative stroke after CABG. (Tarakji, Sabik et al. 2011) In the REACH Registry which was comprised of 67,888 patients, 10% of patients had concomitant coronary artery disease (CAD) and cerebrovascular disease (CVD). Anastasiasdis et al evaluated carotid arteries in 307 patients undergoing CABG and reported that while 3 out of 4 patients undergoing CABG had carotid atherosclerosis, the majority of these (63%) had <

Management of Carotid Artery Disease in the Setting of Coronary Artery Disease in Need of
Coronary Artery Bypass Surgery

81

50% ECAS. (Anastasiadis, Karamitsos et al. 2009). Various studies have reported the incidence of ECAS with varies degree of stenosis among the patient populations undergoing CABG which are summarized in table 1.

Study	Number of patients undergoing CABG being evaluated for ECAS	Prevalence of ECAS %
Wanamaker et al	559	ECAS >50% : 36%
Shirani et al	1045	ECAS > 60% : 6.9%
Anastasiadis et al	307	ECAS > 70% : 13%
Cornily et al	205	ECAS >70% : 5.8%
Salasidis et al	387	ECAS > 80% : 8.5%
Schwartz et al	582	ECAS > 50% . 22% ECAS > 80% : 12%

Abbreviations: CABG, coronary artery bypass grating'; ECAS, extracranial carotid artery stenosis.

Table 1. Prevalence of extracranial carotid artery stenosis among patients undergoing coronary artery bypass grafting.

Salasidis et al identified increasing age, history of previous carotid revascularization and presence of PAD in addition to severe ECAS as risk factors for neurological events after cardiac surgery, highlighting that ECAS is only 1 of a number of factors that drives peri-operative stroke risk.(Salasidis, Latter et al. 1995)

Interestingly, the likelihood of having ECAS increases with the underlying severity of CAD (Table 2).

Severity of CAD	Prevalence of Significant Carotid Atherosclerosis (%)
1- vessel CAD	5.3%
2- vessel CAD	13.5%
3- vessel CAD	24.5%
Left main disease	40%
3-vessel CAD or left main disease	24%

Table 2. Prevalence of significant carotid artery stenosis (extracranial carotid artery stenosis ≥ 50%) among patients with different severity of coronary artery disease based on number of vessels involved or left main disease.

It was postulated that increasing degree of stenosis was associated with increased risk of perioperative stroke by Naylor et al who reported that among 5,453 patients undergoing CABG, the risk of perioperative stroke was <2%, 3%, 5% and 7-11% among patients who had < 50% ECAS, 50-99% unilateral ECAS, 50-99% bilateral ECAS and occluded carotid artery respectively.(Naylor, Mehta et al. 2002)

2. Screening for carotid artery disease

Screening for carotid artery disease is usually performed with carotid duplex ultrasound. Screening recommendations for carotid artery disease are somewhat controversial and vary across medical societies.(Goldstein, Adams et al. 2006; Bates, Babb et al. 2007; Qureshi, Alexandrov et al. 2007; 2008; Brott, Halperin et al. 2011) The most widely accepted multisocietal vascular practice guidelines involving 14 different vascular societies including the American College of Cardiology Foundation, American Heart Association Task Force on Practice Guidelines, the American Stroke Association, American Association of Neuroscience Nurses, American Association of Neurological Surgeons, American College of Radiology, American Society of Neuroradiology, Congress of Neurological Surgeons, Society of Atherosclerosis Imaging and Prevention,Society for Cardiovascular Angiography and Interventions, Society of Interventional Radiology, Society of NeuroInterventional Surgery, Society for Vascular Medicine, and Society for Vascular Surgery recommend screening for patients with carotid bruit or patients with CAD or symptomatic PAD or atherosclerotic aortic aneurysm as well those who may not have evidence of atherosclerosis but have 2 or more cardiovascular risk factors such as hypertension, dyslipidemia, tobacco smoking, family history of premature atherosclerosis or family history of ischemic stroke.(Brott, Halperin et al. 2011). The US Preventive Service Task Force recommended against screening as it was not cost-effective in asymptomatic patients.(Bates, Babb et al. 2007) The American Society of Neuroimaging recommended against the screening of unselected populations but advised the screening of adults older than 65 years of age who have 3 or more cardiovascular risk factors (Qureshi, Alexandrov et al. 2007)

For patients undergoing elective CABG, the multi-societal guidelines recommend screening for carotid artery disease in patients older than 65 years of age and in those with left main stenosis, PAD, history of cigarette smoking, history of stroke or TIA or carotid bruit. The American Heart Association and American College of Cardiology CABG guidelines offer recommendations consistent with the multi-societal vascular guidelines, however they also recommend that patients who have history of hypertension or diabetes mellitus also undergo preoperative carotid duplex scanning.(Hillis, Smith et al. 2011)

3. Utility of advanced imaging carotid artery beyond carotid duplex ultrasound

Duplex ultrasound is an excellent tool to diagnose ECAS.(Eagle, Guyton et al. 1999) However there are certain inherent errors that can occur with duplex. The presence of calcification at the site of stenosis may cause underestimation of degree of stenosis; similarly contralateral occlusion may lead to falsely elevated velocities in the ipsilateral carotid artery leading to overestimation of the degree of stenosis. (Mitchell E 2004) In such situations additional imaging with computed tomography angiography (CTA) or magnetic resonance angiography (MRA) may further characterize the degree of stenosis as well as provide insight on plaque characteristics, aortic pathology and intracranial ICA abnormalities. Given the excellent images rendered by CTA or MRA, conventional angiography is rarely required for determining degree of stenosis among those with normal or minimally impaired renal function. For those with moderate to severe chronic kidney disease, MRI may be relatively contraindicated due to the risk of nephrogenic systemic sclerosis and invasive angiography favored over CTA given its lower relative contrast volume and risk of contrast-induced acute kidney injury.

Other factors that may lead to increased stroke risk beyond degree of stenosis, including cerebrovascular reserve (CVR). Severe ECAS reduces cerebral perfusion pressure. Autoregulation of the cerebral vasculature dilates the cerebral arterioles maximally, and with further reduction in cerebral perfusion, blood flow will eventually decrease, causing impairment in cerebral perfusion leading to stroke. CVR can be assessed by two approaches. the first, CVR can be determined through direct measurements of brain tissue with flow-sensitive imaging through positron emission tomography, CT perfusion or MR perfusion before and after vasodilator stimulation. A second, indirect approach utilizes transcranial Doppler to assess flow velocities distal to the lesion, typically in the middle cerebral artery before and after vasodilatory stimulation, with increase in flow velocities used to indirectly measure CVR. (Gupta, Chazen et al. 2012) In a meta-analysis of patients with severe ECAS, there was an association between impaired CVR and increased stroke risk.(Gupta, Chazen et al. 2012) An incomplete circle of Willis has also been associated with increased ipsilateral cerebral ischemia during carotid cross clamping with CEA.(Manninen, Makinen et al. 2009) and as a risk factor for ischemic stroke (Hoksbergen AW et al. Cerebrovasc Dz 2003;16:191-8) Current guidelines do not comment on use of cerebral perfusion imaging when assessing stroke risk due to insufficient evidence available so far.(Brott, Halperin et al. 2011; Hillis, Smith et al. 2011)

4. Treatment

Treatment options for ECAS consist of medical therapy and in some cases, revascularization.

Medical therapy for carotid artery disease: Medical therapy is the cornerstone of treatment for atherosclerotic disease. Medical therapy for ECAS comprises of treatment of risk factors such as hypertension, dyslipidemia, diabetes mellitus, and tobacco use and use of antiplatelet therapy. Consensus societal class I recommendations for treatment of atherosclerotic carotid artery disease appear in Table 1 (Brott, Halperin et al. 2011).

Treatment of hypertension: Hypertension increases risk of stroke significantly. For each 10 mm Hg rise in blood pressure, the stroke risk increases by 30 to 45%. This risk significantly is significantly reduced with antihypertensive therapy. A systemic review of 7 randomized controlled trials (RCT) showed that treatment with antihypertensive agents reduced the risk of recurrent stroke by 24%. A meta-analysis of 40 studies with > 188,000 patients reported a 33% decreased risk of stroke with a 10 mm Hg reduction in BP.(Lawes, Bennett et al. 2004; Brott, Halperin et al. 2011) Hypertension should be treated to maintain a goal blood pressure (BP) < 140/90 mm Hg for all patients with ECAS except those with diabetes mellitus (DM) and chronic

Recommendation	Class of Indication	Level of Evidence
Antihypertensive treatment is recommended for patients with hypertension and asymptomatic extracranial carotid or vertebral atherosclerosis to maintain blood pressure below 140/90 mm Hg	I	A
Treatment with a statin medication is recommended for all patients with extracranial carotid or vertebral atherosclerosis to reduce low-density lipoprotein (LDL) cholesterol below 100 mg/dL	I	B
Patients with extracranial carotid or vertebral atherosclerosis who smoke cigarettes should be advised to quit smoking and offered smoking cessation interventions to reduce the risks of atherosclerosis progression and stroke	I	B
Antiplatelet therapy with aspirin, 75 to 325 mg daily, is recommended for patients with obstructive or nonobstructive atherosclerosis that involves the extracranial carotid and/or vertebral arteries for prevention of MI and other ischemic cardiovascular events, although the benefit has not been established for prevention of stroke in asymptomatic patients	I	A
In patients with obstructive or nonobstructive extracranial carotid or vertebral atherosclerosis who have sustained ischemic stroke or TIA, antiplatelet therapy with aspirin alone (75 to 325 mg daily), clopidogrel alone (75 mg daily), or the combination of aspirin plus extended-release dipyridamole (25 and 200 mg twice daily, respectively) is recommended (*Level of Evidence: B*) and preferred over the combination of aspirin with clopidogrel	I	B
Aspirin (81 to 325 mg daily) is recommended before CEA and may be continued indefinitely postoperatively	I	A
Beyond the first month after CEA, aspirin (75 to 325 mg daily), clopidogrel (75 mg daily), or the combination of low-dose aspirin plus extended-release dipyridamole (25 and 200 mg twice daily, respectively) should be administered for long-term prophylaxis against ischemic cardiovascular events	I	B
Administration of antihypertensive medication is recommended as needed to control blood pressure before and after CEA.	I	C
The findings on clinical neurological examination should be documented within 24 hours before and after CEA.	I	C
Before and for a minimum of 30 days after CAS, dual-antiplatelet therapy with aspirin (81 to 325 mg daily) plus clopidogrel (75 mg daily) is recommended. For patients intolerant of clopidogrel, ticlopidine (250 mg twice daily) may be substituted.	I	C
Administration of antihypertensive medication is recommended to control blood pressure before and after CAS.	I	C

Table 3. Recommendations from multisocietal guidelines for extracranial carotid artery stenosis.

kidney disease (CKD) in whom goal BP is < 130/80 mm Hg.(Chobanian, Bakris et al. 2003). These guidelines are applicable to all patients except those in the hyperacute period after stroke. The type of agent utilized should be based on presence of other co-morbid conditions (e.g., diabetes, CKD, CAD, etc.) and not on presence of carotid disease.(Chobanian, Bakris et al. 2003).

Management of Diabetes Mellitus: Presence of diabetes mellitus is associated with increased stroke risk. In the Rotterdam study, diabetes was the only risk factor independently associated with severe progression of carotid stenosis.(van der Meer, Iglesias del Sol et al. 2003). Although glycemic control is necessary, intensive control may not be of incremental benefit. In the UKPDS study, intensive glucose control compared to conventional glucose control did not reduce stroke risk. Similarly, in the ACCORD and ADVANCE trials, intensive glucose control to lower hemoglobin A1c <6 or <6.5, respectively, did not reduce stroke risk when compared to conventional treatment.(Gerstein, Miller et al. 2008; Patel, MacMahon et al. 2008) Intensive control of other risk factors in patients with diabetes is also beneficial, such as administering statins in patients with diabetes even with 'normal' serum cholesterol. Doing so may lower the risk of stroke by as much as 48%.(Colhoun, Betteridge et al. 2004). All diabetic patients with atherosclerotic ECAS should be treated with diet, exercise and glucose lowering drugs as needed to maintain hemoglobin A1c <7. All patients should be treated with statins regardless of cholesterol levels and LDL cholesterol goal should be < 100mg/dl.(Brott, Halperin et al. 2011)

Treatment of dyslipidemia: Dyslipidemia isn't as strongly associated with ischemic stroke as hypertension or diabetes mellitus. In the MR-FIT trial which involved over 350,000 men, the relative risk of death was 2.5 times higher in men with highest vs. the lowest cholesterol levels. (Iso, Jacobs et al. 1989) In the ARIC study, dyslipidemia weakly correlated with ischemic stroke. (Shahar, Chambless et al. 2003); however in the Women's Health Study which evaluated over 27,000 women, total and LDL cholesterol were associated with increased risk of stroke.(Kurth, Everett et al. 2007). The lipid lowering agents of choice are the statins which in addition to lowering cholesterol, work through so-called provide pleotropic effects such as plaque stabilization and reduction in inflammation which may help reduce overall cardiovascular events. A metanalysis comprising of 26 trials with > 90,000 patients found that statins reduce stroke risk by 21%; With every 10% reduction of serum LDL cholesterol, there was a 15.6% reduction in stroke.(Amarenco, Labreuche et al. 2004). The SPARCL trial randomized patients with recent stroke or TIA to atorvastatin 80 mg daily or placebo and found that atorvastatin reduced the incidence of ischemic stroke by 22%.(Amarenco, Bogousslavsky et al. 2006) All patients with atherosclerotic carotid artery disease should be treated with statin to maintain an LDL cholesterol < 100 mg/dl and it is reasonable to maintain LDL cholesterol < 70 mg/dl, especially in high risk patients such as those with ECAS and one or more cardiac risk factors such as current smoker or diabetes mellitus. If the goal LDL cholesterol is not achieved with statin therapy, other lipid lowering agents such as bile acid sequestrants, niacin or ezetimibe can be added to statin therapy.(Brott, Halperin et al. 2011)

Smoking Cessation: Smoking is strongly associated with increased stroke risk. Cigarette smoking is associated with 50% increase in relative risk of ischemic stroke.(Howard, Wagenknecht et al. 1998) Even patients who are past cigarette smokers have a 25% higher risk of stroke compared to lifelong non-smokers.(Howard, Wagenknecht et al. 1998) The Framingham

Heart Study and Cardiovascular Health Study both have reported an association between quantity and period of time an individual smoked and increased risk of stroke.(Tell, Rutan et al. 1994; Wilson, Hoeg et al. 1997). All smokers should be asked about smoking status on every visit and if currently smoking should be counseled on every visit. Every vascular specialist should assist these patients in developing a plan to quit smoking which would include behavioral and pharmacological interventions.(Rooke, Hirsch et al. 2012)

Antiplatelet therapy: Patients undergoing CABG should be on antiplatelet therapy regardless of the presence or absence of ECAS. The benefits of antiplatelet therapy are well-defined in patients with symptomatic ECAS. (2002), and it appears that clopidogrel is superior to aspirin in preventing death, MI or stroke among those with a history of PAD (CAPRIE PAD subgroup analysis/paper). The benefit of dual antiplatelet therapy over monotherapy in this sub-group of patients is not as well-defined and was not proven in the MATCH or in the overall CHA-RISMA trial.(Diener, Bogousslavsky et al. 2004; Bhatt, Fox et al. 2006) However, in the CHARISMA trial, dual antiplatelet therapy with aspirin and clopidogrel did reduce the incidence of death, MI or stroke among those with established atherosclerotic vascular disease at baseline.(Bhatt, Fox et al. 2006). The ESPS-2 trial demonstrated that extended-release dipyridamale 200 mg twice daily along with aspirin 25 mg once daily (aggrenox) was superior to aspirin alone in secondary prevention of ischemic strokes.(Diener, Cunha et al. 1996) The PROFESS trial compared aggrenox to clopidogrel for secondary prevention of ischemic stroke and found no difference in recurrent stroke reduction in both groups.(Sacco, Diener et al. 2008). Anticoagulant therapy was evaluated in the WARSS study where aspirin was compared to warfarin for stroke prevention in patients with recent stroke, No added benefit was observed with warfarin compared to aspirin in patients with large-vessel atherosclerosis.(Mohr, Thompson et al. 2001). Patients undergoing CABG who have atherosclerotic ECAS will benefit from antiplatelet monotherapy with at aspirin at a minimum; whether dual antiplatelet therapy is incrementally beneficial is less well established.

In summary, it is recommended that all patients with ECAS, regardless of whether they are to undergo CABG receive aggressive risk factor modification in addition to statins, beta-blockers, angiotensin converting enzyme inhibitors or angiotensin receptor blockers and antiplatelet therapy unless contraindicated.

Revascularization: The overall goal of carotid artery revascularization is to reduce the incidence of stroke beyond that afforded by medical therapy alone. In the perioperative setting, the decision about whether to perform carotid artery revascularization, which revasculariza-tion modality to pursue and when to revascularize (e.g., CEA or CAS preceded by CABG, CABG preceded by CEA or CAS, concomitant CEA or CAS at the time of CABG). remain challenging.

Indications for carotid revascularization: The decision to revascularize the carotid artery hinges on the presence or absence of symptoms attributable to ECAS, degree of ECAS and urgency of CABG.

The current multisocietal vascular guidelines recommend that carotid revascularization by CEA or CAS with embolic protection before or concurrent with myocardial revascularization surgery is reasonable in patients with greater than 80% carotid stenosis who have experienced ipsilateral retinal or hemispheric cerebral ischemic symptoms within 6 months. They also state that in patients with asymptomatic carotid stenosis, even if severe, the safety and efficacy of carotid revascularization before or concurrent with myocardial revascularization are not well established..(Brott, Halperin et al. 2011)

The American College of Cardiology and American Heart Association CABG guidelines state that is reasonable to revascularize ECAS of 50-99% in patients with previous history of stroke or TIA and In those who do not have a prior history of stroke or TIA, they consider it reasonable to revascularize especially in the setting of bilateral ECAS of 70-99% or unilateral ECAS of 70-99% with contralateral occlusion. (Hillis, Smith et al. 2011)

In addition to it is necessary to identify and appropriately treat other factors such as atrial fibrillation, low output cardiac state, aortic arch atheroma, age, diabetes etc which also increase the risk for perioperative stroke.

Strategies for carotid revascularization in patients undergoing CABG:

The 2 revascularization modalities most commonly used are CEA and carotid stenting. Both of these modalities are approved by the Food and Drug Administration (FDA) for carotid revascularization. (FDA 2011)

Carotid endarterectomy: CEA has proven to beneficial in stroke reduction in patients with symptomatic and asymptomatic ECAS.(1991; 1991; 1995; 1996; 1998; Barnett, Taylor et al. 1998; Halliday, Mansfield et al. 2004; Halliday, Harrison et al. 2010)

There are three surgical strategies for carotid revascularization in patients undergoing CABG:

Concomitant CEA-CABG: CEA is performed prior CABG under the same anesthesia.

"Staged CEA- CABG": CEA is performed prior to CABG in different settings. Patient is initially schedule for CEA and then later for CABG,

"Reverse staged": Here CABG is initially performed and then CEA is scheduled at a later date or time.

A meta-analysis of 56 reports comparing these 3 surgical strategies showed higher rates of stroke in patients undergoing reverse staged procedures (10%) as compared to concomitant (6%) and staged procedures (5%) However, staged procedures had the highest rates of perioperative MI (11%[p=0.01]) and death (9%[p=0.02]) compared to concomitant(5% & 6%) and reverse staged procedures (3% and 4%).(Moore, Barnett et al. 1995) Another meta-analysis of 16 studies with over 800 concomitant and 920 staged procedures showed a increased risk of composite endpoint of stroke or death among patients undergoing combined procedure compared to staged procedures (9.5% v 5.7%; relative risk 1.49; 95% confidence interval 1.03-2.15; p = 0.034).(Borger, Fremes et al. 1999) Naylor et al performed a systematic review comparing outcomes following staged or concomitant procedures which included 94 studies with concomitant procedures and 24 studies with staged procedures.(Naylor, Cuffe et al. 2003) 60% of the patients in these studies were asymptomatic. Bilateral 50-99% ECAS or carotid occlusion was present in 30-37% of the patients. Thirty nine % of patient who underwent concomitant were labeled as having "urgent" surgery, 72% of them were classified as having New York Heart Association grade 3 or 4 and 25% of patients had left main disease.(Naylor, Cuffe et al. 2003) It was noted that mortality was highest among the patients undergoing concomitant (4.6%, 95% CI 4.1-5.2) and death ± stroke rate was also higher compared to other staged procedure (8.7%, 95% CI 7.7-9.8). Reverse staged procedures had the highest risk of ipsilateral stroke (5.8%, 95% CI 0.0-14.3) and any stroke (6.3%, 95% CI 1.0-11.7) but with the lowest risk for peri-operative MI (0.9%, 95% CI 0.5-1.4). Staged procedures had the lowest rate of death ± stroke (6.1%, 95% CI 2.9-9.3) but the highest rate of peri-operative MI (6.5%, 95% CI 3.2-9.7). However, the benefit seen with staged procedures on reduction in stroke and death was no longer significant when peri-operative MI was also included in the combined outcomes. The risk of death/stroke/ MI was 11.5% (95% CI 10.1-12.9) following concomitant procedures versus 10.2% (95% CI 7.4-13.1) after staged procedures. Non of these studies had randomized patients to the different strategies and hence may have selection bias.

Carotid Artery Stenting: Randomized clinical trials have shown that carotid stenting is an effective method of revascularization equivalent to carotid endarterectomy.(Yadav, Wholey et al. 2004; Brott, Hobson et al. 2010) The protected carotid-artery stenting versus endarterectomy in high-risk patients (SAFFIRE) trial proved efficacy of carotid stenting. It consisted of patients at high surgical risk who were randomized to carotid stenting with embolic protection device or carotid endarterectomy. The study proved that carotid stenting was non-inferior to CEA (cumulative incidence, 20.1 percent; absolute difference, -7.9 percentage points; 95 percent confidence interval, -16.4 to 0.7 percentage points; P=0.004 for noninferiority, and P=0.053 for superiority). (Massop, Dave et al. 2009) Sixteen percent of patients in the SAFFIRE trial had severe CAD too. In the Stenting versus Endarterectomy for Treatment of Carotid-Artery Stenosis (CREST) trial, 2502 patients with indication for carotid revascularization were randomized to carotid stenting or CEA regardless of level of surgical risk. The CREST showed that CAS had similar adverse outcomes as CEA proving it to be equivalent to CEA for revascularization (7.2% and 6.8%, respectively; hazard ratio with stenting, 1.11; 95% confidence interval, 0.81 to 1.51; P=0.51).(Brott, Hobson et al. 2010).

Three different strategies can be utilized when carotid stenting is performed in patients undergoing CABG:

1. "Staged": CAS followed by CABG (CABG is done weeks later after CAS)

2. "Same day hybrid": CAS followed by CABG on the same day.

3. Concomitant ("true hybrid"): CAS followed by CABG on the same day in the same OR done immediately after CAS is completed.

In the staged method after carotid stenting, patients are treated with dual antiplatelet therapy with aspirin and clopidogrel for a few weeks (most commonly 4 weeks). Later, clopidogrel is held for 5-7 days prior to CABG. Patients undergoing hybrid procedures (true or same day) are placed on heparin between procedures and later on clopidogrel as soon as possible after CABG.

Mendiz et al reported 30 high surgical risk patients for CEA who underwent synchronous CAS then CABG and/or valve surgery. Among these patients, 1 patient had TIA and no patients suffered stroke or MI.(Mendiz, Fava et al. 2006) Versaci et al reported 101 patients who underwent CABG immediately after CAS. The 30-day composite incidence of disabling stroke, AMI or death was 4%: 2 patients had stroke after CAS. (Versaci, Reimers et al. 2009). Another series of 22 patients who underwent true hybrid procedure showed no deaths or MI and one case of contralateral stroke. There were no cases of major postoperative bleeding or stent thrombosis.(Palombo, Stella et al. 2009) Van der Heyden et al reported 356 patients with asymptomatic ECAS who underwent staged CAS - CABG with a mean interval of 22 days between the 2 procedures. The 30-day post-CABG stroke and death rate was 4.8%, MI was 2% and MI and death was 6.7%.(Van der Heyden, Suttorp et al. 2007) Naylor et al performed a meta-analysis of 11 studies involving 760 CAS plus CABG procedures.(Naylor, Mehta et al. 2009) Majority of the patients in this analysis were asymptomatic (87%) and majority had unilateral ECAS (82%). The study reported a mortality of 5.5% (95% confidence interval, CI: 3.4-7.6), ipsilateral stroke rate of 3.3% (95% CI: 1.6-5.1), all-cause stroke rate of 4.2% (95% CI: 2.4-6.1) and a MI rate of 1.8% (95% CI: 0.5-3.0) at 30-day follow-up. These results are comparable to systematic reviews of staged and concomitant carotid CEA-CABG, and suggest that staged CAS-CABG appears to as effective as staged CEA-CABG.

Decision regarding appropriate procedure and strategy for carotid revascularization in patients with undergoing CABG:

There are no randomized clinical trials comparing CAS and CEA in this patient group. Data from the Nationwide Inpatient Sample consisting of 27,084 patients who underwent carotid stenting before CABG or combined CEA - CABG surgery during the 5 years from 2000 to 2004 reported that 96.7% underwent CEA plus CABG surgery versus 3.3% who had carotid stenting plus CABG. Fewer perioperative strokes were reported among patients undergoing staged carotid stenting - CABG than among those undergoing staged CEA - CABG stroke (2.4% versus 3.9%). In this non-randomized data, patients undergoing staged CEA - CABG surgery faced a 62% greater risk of postoperative stroke than patients undergoing staged CAS-CABG surgery (OR 1.62, 95% CI 1.1 to 2.5; p<0.02).(Timaran, Rosero et al. 2008) There was no difference in the combined risk of stroke and death between the treatment (OR 1.26, 95% CI 0.9 to 1.6; p=NS).(Timaran, Rosero et al. 2008) Another study compared hybrid CAS - CABG procedures (n=56) to concomitant CEA-CABG procedure (n=111). In this study patients undergoing CAS at baseline were more likely to have unstable/severe angina (52% vs 27%, p = 0.002), severe left ventricular dysfunction (20% vs. 9%, p = 0.05), symptomatic carotid disease (46% vs. 23%, p = 0.002), and the need for repeat open heart surgery (32% vs. 9%, p = 0.0002). Severe contra-lateral carotid disease was more prevalent in the concomitant CEA+CABG group (28% vs. 11%, p = 0.01). On 30-day follow-up, CAS group had a significantly lower incidence of stroke or MI (5% vs. 19%, p = 0.02). (Ziada, Yadav et al. 2005) Another study involving 659 patients in whom CEA-CABG, CAS–CABG (staged) or CAS-CABG (hybrid) was performed in 28.1%, 57.4% and 13.5% of patients respectively showed a 30-day composite endpoint of death, MI and stroke of 4.8%, 2.4% and 8.6% respectively (p=0.01). (Ribichini, Tomai et al. 2010)

Timing of carotid revascularization when indicated is chosen based on symptoms status of the carotid and coronary territory, severity of carotid and coronary disease and level of expertise available at the institution.(Venkatachalam and Shishehbor 2011)

Symptomatic carotid artery disease with ECAS >50-99% stenosis:

1. Symptomatic carotid disease and asymptomatic coronary disease or stable angina: In these patients carotid revascularization should be pursued prior to CABG, staged carotid stenting then followed by 4 weeks of dual antiplatelet and then CABG or staged CEA - CABG or concomitant CEA-CABD is usually considered. Selection of patients for carotid stenting or CEA is based co-morbidities, anatomy and local expertise available.

2. Symptomatic carotid disease and symptomatic coronary disease (acute coronary syndromes): In these patients carotid disease should be revascularized initially or concomitantly. Concomitant CEA-CABG or "same day" or "true hybrid" stenting procedures are usually considered. In case need for emergent CABG's, reverse stages CABG-CEA procedures can be considered.

Asymptomatic carotid stenosis (ECAS> 80-99%) is further classified as high risk or low risk groups. High risk group consists of patients with bilateral ECAS > 80-99% or unilateral ECAS >80-99% with contralateral occlusion and asymptomatic ECAS 80-99% with impaired cerebral perfusion reserve. Patients without these features are considered low risk.

1. Asymptomatic ECAS with high risk features and symptomatic coronary disease (acute coronary syndromes): These patients are at high risk for myocardial infarction as well as stroke and hence should be considered for concomitant CEA-CABG or "same day" or "true hybrid" CAS-CABG.

2. Asymptomatic ECAS with high risk features with stable angina: These patients should be considered for staged CAS-CABG.

3. Asymptomatic ECAS with low risk features and stable angina or acute coronary syndromes: These patents should initially undergo coronary revascularization with carotid revascularization (stenting or CEA) at a later date on an elective basis.

5. Conclusion

To date, stroke remains one of the most devastating complications after open heart surgery with serious adverse economic, psychological and clinical implications on healthcare and individuals suffering from it.(Roach, Kanchuger et al. 1996; Hogue, Murphy et al. 1999) Identifying patients at risk of stroke after CABG and applying measures to reduce its occurrence are extremely vital.

Management of Carotid Artery Disease in the Setting of Coronary Artery Disease in Need of
Coronary Artery Bypass Surgery

91

Author details

Aditya M. Sharma[1] and Herbert D. Aronow[2]

1 University of Virginia, Charlottesville, VA, USA

2 St. Joseph Mercy Hospital, Ann Arbor MI, USA

References

[1] (1991). "Beneficial effect of carotid endarterectomy in symptomatic patients with high-grade carotid stenosis. North American Symptomatic Carotid Endarterectomy Trial Collaborators." *N Engl J Med* 325(7): 445-453.

[2] (1991). "MRC European Carotid Surgery Trial: interim results for symptomatic patients with severe (70-99%) or with mild (0-29%) carotid stenosis. European Carotid Surgery Trialists' Collaborative Group." *Lancet* 337(8752): 1235-1243.

[3] (1995). "Endarterectomy for asymptomatic carotid artery stenosis. Executive Committee for the Asymptomatic Carotid Atherosclerosis Study." *JAMA* 273(18): 1421-1428.

[4] (1996). "Endarterectomy for moderate symptomatic carotid stenosis: interim results from the MRC European Carotid Surgery Trial." *Lancet* 347(9015): 1591-1593.

[5] (1998). "Randomised trial of endarterectomy for recently symptomatic carotid stenosis: final results of the MRC European Carotid Surgery Trial (ECST)." *Lancet* 351(9113): 1379-1387.

[6] (2002). "Collaborative meta-analysis of randomised trials of antiplatelet therapy for prevention of death, myocardial infarction, and stroke in high risk patients." *BMJ* 324(7329): 71-86.

[7] (2008). "Screening for carotid artery stenosis: recommendation statement." *Am Fam Physician* 77(7): 1006-1010.

[8] Amarenco, P., J. Bogousslavsky, et al. (2006). "High-dose atorvastatin after stroke or transient ischemic attack." *N Engl J Med* 355(6): 549-559.

[9] Amarenco, P., J. Labreuche, et al. (2004). "Statins in stroke prevention and carotid atherosclerosis: systematic review and up-to-date meta-analysis." *Stroke* 35(12): 2902-2909.

[10] Anastasiadis, K., T. D. Karamitsos, et al. (2009). "Preoperative screening and management of carotid artery disease in patients undergoing cardiac surgery." *Perfusion* 24(4): 257-262.

[11] Barnett, H. J., D. W. Taylor, et al. (1998). "Benefit of carotid endarterectomy in pa-
      tients with symptomatic moderate or severe stenosis. North American Symptomatic
      Carotid Endarterectomy Trial Collaborators." N Engl J Med 339(20): 1415-1425.

[12] Bates, E. R., J. D. Babb, et al. (2007). "ACCF/SCAI/SVMB/SIR/ASITN 2007 clinical ex-
      pert consensus document on carotid stenting: a report of the American College of
      Cardiology Foundation Task Force on Clinical Expert Consensus Documents (ACCF/
      SCAI/SVMB/SIR/ASITN Clinical Expert Consensus Document Committee on Carotid
      Stenting)." J Am Coll Cardiol 49(1): 126-170.

[13] Beique, F., M. Ali, et al. (2006). "Canadian guidelines for training in adult periopera-
      tive transesophageal echocardiography. Recommendations of the Cardiovascular
      Section of the Canadian Anesthesiologists' Society and the Canadian Society of Echo-
      cardiography." Can J Cardiol 22(12): 1015-1027.

[14] Bhatt, D. L., K. A. Fox, et al. (2006). "Clopidogrel and aspirin versus aspirin alone for
      the prevention of atherothrombotic events." N Engl J Med 354(16): 1706-1717.

[15] Borger, M. A., S. E. Fremes, et al. (1999). "Coronary bypass and carotid endarterecto-
      my: does a combined approach increase risk? A metaanalysis." Ann Thorac Surg 68(1):
      14-20; discussion 21.

[16] Brott, T. G., J. L. Halperin, et al. (2011). "2011 ASA/ACCF/AHA/AANN/AANS/ACR/
      ASNR/CNS/SAIP/SCAI/SIR/SNIS/SVM/SVS guideline on the management of pa-
      tients with extracranial carotid and vertebral artery disease. A report of the American
      College of Cardiology Foundation/American Heart Association Task Force on Prac-
      tice Guidelines, and the American Stroke Association, American Association of Neu-
      roscience Nurses, American Association of Neurological Surgeons, American College
      of Radiology, American Society of Neuroradiology, Congress of Neurological Sur-
      geons, Society of Atherosclerosis Imaging and Prevention, Society for Cardiovascular
      Angiography and Interventions, Society of Interventional Radiology, Society of Neu-
      roInterventional Surgery, Society for Vascular Medicine, and Society for Vascular
      Surgery." Circulation 124(4): e54-130.

[17] Brott, T. G., J. L. Halperin, et al. (2011). "2011 ASA/ACCF/AHA/AANN/AANS/ACR/
      ASNR/CNS/SAIP/SCAI/SIR/SNIS/SVM/SVS guideline on the management of pa-
      tients with extracranial carotid and vertebral artery disease: executive summary. A
      report of the American College of Cardiology Foundation/American Heart Associa-
      tion Task Force on Practice Guidelines, and the American Stroke Association, Ameri-
      can Association of Neuroscience Nurses, American Association of Neurological
      Surgeons, American College of Radiology, American Society of Neuroradiology,
      Congress of Neurological Surgeons, Society of Atherosclerosis Imaging and Preven-
      tion, Society for Cardiovascular Angiography and Interventions, Society of Interven-
      tional Radiology, Society of NeuroInterventional Surgery, Society for Vascular
      Medicine, and Society for Vascular Surgery." Circulation 124(4): 489-532.

[18] Brott, T. G., J. L. Halperin, et al. (2011). "2011 ASA/ACCF/AHA/AANN/AANS/ACR/
      ASNR/CNS/SAIP/SCAI/SIR/SNIS/SVM/SVS guideline on the management of pa-

tients with extracranial carotid and vertebral artery disease: executive summary. A report of the American College of Cardiology Foundation/American Heart Association Task Force on Practice Guidelines, and the American Stroke Association, American Association of Neuroscience Nurses, American Association of Neurological Surgeons, American College of Radiology, American Society of Neuroradiology, Congress of Neurological Surgeons, Society of Atherosclerosis Imaging and Prevention, Society for Cardiovascular Angiography and Interventions, Society of Interventional Radiology, Society of NeuroInterventional Surgery, Society for Vascular Medicine, and Society for Vascular Surgery." *Circulation* 124(4): 489-532.

[19] Brott, T. G., R. W. Hobson, 2nd, et al. (2010). "Stenting versus endarterectomy for treatment of carotid-artery stenosis." *N Engl J Med* 363(1): 11-23.

[20] Brown, P. P., A. D. Kugelmass, et al. (2008). "The frequency and cost of complications associated with coronary artery bypass grafting surgery: results from the United States Medicare program." *Ann Thorac Surg* 85(6): 1980-1986.

[21] Chobanian, A. V., G. L. Bakris, et al. (2003). "The Seventh Report of the Joint National Committee on Prevention, Detection, Evaluation, and Treatment of High Blood Pressure: the JNC 7 report." *JAMA* 289(19): 2560-2572.

[22] Colhoun, H. M., D. J. Betteridge, et al. (2004). "Primary prevention of cardiovascular disease with atorvastatin in type 2 diabetes in the Collaborative Atorvastatin Diabetes Study (CARDS): multicentre randomised placebo-controlled trial." *Lancet* 364(9435): 685-696.

[23] Diener, H. C., J. Bogousslavsky, et al. (2004). "Aspirin and clopidogrel compared with clopidogrel alone after recent ischaemic stroke or transient ischaemic attack in high-risk patients (MATCH): randomised, double-blind, placebo-controlled trial." *Lancet* 364(9431): 331-337.

[24] Diener, H. C., L. Cunha, et al. (1996). "European Stroke Prevention Study. 2. Dipyridamole and acetylsalicylic acid in the secondary prevention of stroke." *J Neurol Sci* 143(1-2): 1-13.

[25] Eagle, K. A., R. A. Guyton, et al. (1999). "ACC/AHA guidelines for coronary artery bypass graft surgery: executive summary and recommendations : A report of the American College of Cardiology/American Heart Association Task Force on Practice Guidelines (Committee to revise the 1991 guidelines for coronary artery bypass graft surgery)." *Circulation* 100(13): 1464-1480.

[26] FDA. (2011). "http://www.fda.gov/NewsEvents/Newsroom/PressAnnouncements/ucm254430.htm."

[27] Furlan, A. J., C. A. Sila, et al. (1992). "Neurologic complications related to cardiac surgery." *Neurol Clin* 10(1): 145-166.

[28] Gerstein, H. C., M. E. Miller, et al. (2008). "Effects of intensive glucose lowering in type 2 diabetes." *N Engl J Med* 358(24): 2545-2559.

[29] Go, A. S., D. Mozaffarian, et al. (2012). "Heart Disease and Stroke Statistics--2013 Update A Report From the American Heart Association." *Circulation.*

[30] Goldstein, L. B., R. Adams, et al. (2006). "Primary prevention of ischemic stroke: a guideline from the American Heart Association/American Stroke Association Stroke Council: cosponsored by the Atherosclerotic Peripheral Vascular Disease Interdisciplinary Working Group; Cardiovascular Nursing Council; Clinical Cardiology Council; Nutrition, Physical Activity, and Metabolism Council; and the Quality of Care and Outcomes Research Interdisciplinary Working Group: the American Academy of Neurology affirms the value of this guideline." *Stroke* 37(6): 1583-1633.

[31] Gupta, A., J. L. Chazen, et al. (2012). "Cerebrovascular reserve and stroke risk in patients with carotid stenosis or occlusion: a systematic review and meta-analysis." *Stroke* 43(11): 2884-2891.

[32] Halliday, A., M. Harrison, et al. (2010). "10-year stroke prevention after successful carotid endarterectomy for asymptomatic stenosis (ACST-1): a multicentre randomised trial." *Lancet* 376(9746): 1074-1084.

[33] Halliday, A., A. Mansfield, et al. (2004). "Prevention of disabling and fatal strokes by successful carotid endarterectomy in patients without recent neurological symptoms: randomised controlled trial." *Lancet* 363(9420): 1491-1502.

[34] Hillis, L. D., P. K. Smith, et al. (2011). "2011 ACCF/AHA Guideline for Coronary Artery Bypass Graft Surgery: executive summary: a report of the American College of Cardiology Foundation/American Heart Association Task Force on Practice Guidelines." *Circulation* 124(23): 2610-2642.

[35] Hogue, C. W., Jr., S. F. Murphy, et al. (1999). "Risk factors for early or delayed stroke after cardiac surgery." *Circulation* 100(6): 642-647.

[36] Howard, G., L. E. Wagenknecht, et al. (1998). "Cigarette smoking and other risk factors for silent cerebral infarction in the general population." *Stroke* 29(5): 913-917.

[37] Iso, H., D. R. Jacobs, Jr., et al. (1989). "Serum cholesterol levels and six-year mortality from stroke in 350,977 men screened for the multiple risk factor intervention trial." *N Engl J Med* 320(14): 904-910.

[38] Kallikazaros, I., C. Tsioufis, et al. (1999). "Carotid artery disease as a marker for the presence of severe coronary artery disease in patients evaluated for chest pain." *Stroke* 30(5): 1002-1007.

[39] Kurth, T., B. M. Everett, et al. (2007). "Lipid levels and the risk of ischemic stroke in women." *Neurology* 68(8): 556-562.

[40] Lawes, C. M., D. A. Bennett, et al. (2004). "Blood pressure and stroke: an overview of published reviews." *Stroke* 35(4): 1024.

[41] Manninen, H., K. Makinen, et al. (2009). "How often does an incomplete circle of Willis predispose to cerebral ischemia during closure of carotid artery? Postmortem and clinical imaging studies." *Acta Neurochir (Wien)* 151(9): 1099-1105.

[42] Massop, D., R. Dave, et al. (2009). "Stenting and angioplasty with protection in patients at high-risk for endarterectomy: SAPPHIRE Worldwide Registry first 2,001 patients." *Catheter Cardiovasc Interv* 73(2): 129-136.

[43] Mendiz, O., C. Fava, et al. (2006). "Synchronous carotid stenting and cardiac surgery: an initial single-center experience." *Catheter Cardiovasc Interv* 68(3): 424-428.

[44] Mitchell E, M. G., Zwiebel W, Pellerito J (2004). *Introduction to Vascular Ultrasonography*. Philadelphia, Elsevier.

[45] Mohr, J. P., J. L. Thompson, et al. (2001). "A comparison of warfarin and aspirin for the prevention of recurrent ischemic stroke." *N Engl J Med* 345(20): 1444-1451.

[46] Moore, W. S., H. J. Barnett, et al. (1995). "Guidelines for carotid endarterectomy. A multidisciplinary consensus statement from the ad hoc Committee, American Heart Association." *Stroke* 26(1): 188-201.

[47] Naylor, A. R., R. L. Cuffe, et al. (2003). "A systematic review of outcomes following staged and synchronous carotid endarterectomy and coronary artery bypass." *Eur J Vasc Endovasc Surg* 25(5): 380-389.

[48] Naylor, A. R., Z. Mehta, et al. (2009). "A systematic review and meta-analysis of 30-day outcomes following staged carotid artery stenting and coronary bypass." *Eur J Vasc Endovasc Surg* 37(4): 379-387.

[49] Naylor, A. R., Z. Mehta, et al. (2002). "Carotid artery disease and stroke during coronary artery bypass: a critical review of the literature." *Eur J Vasc Endovasc Surg* 23(4): 283-294.

[50] Palombo, G., N. Stella, et al. (2009). "Safety and effectiveness of combining carotid artery stenting with cardiac surgery: preliminary results of a single-center experience." *J Cardiovasc Surg (Torino)* 50(1): 49-54.

[51] Patel, A., S. MacMahon, et al. (2008). "Intensive blood glucose control and vascular outcomes in patients with type 2 diabetes." *N Engl J Med* 358(24): 2560-2572.

[52] Qureshi, A. I., A. V. Alexandrov, et al. (2007). "Guidelines for screening of extracranial carotid artery disease: a statement for healthcare professionals from the multidisciplinary practice guidelines committee of the American Society of Neuroimaging; cosponsored by the Society of Vascular and Interventional Neurology." *J Neuroimaging* 17(1): 19-47.

[53] Qureshi, A. I., A. V. Alexandrov, et al. (2007). "Guidelines for screening of extracranial carotid artery disease: a statement for healthcare professionals from the multidisci-

plinary practice guidelines committee of the American Society of Neuroimaging; cosponsored by the Society of Vascular and Interventional Neurology." *J Neuroimaging* 17(1): 19-47.

[54] Ribichini, F., F. Tomai, et al. (2010). "Clinical outcome after endovascular, surgical or hybrid revascularisation in patients with combined carotid and coronary artery disease: the Finalised Research In ENDovascular Strategies Study Group (FRIENDS)." *EuroIntervention* 6(3): 328-335.

[55] Roach, G. W., M. Kanchuger, et al. (1996). "Adverse cerebral outcomes after coronary bypass surgery. Multicenter Study of Perioperative Ischemia Research Group and the Ischemia Research and Education Foundation Investigators." *N Engl J Med* 335(25): 1857-1863.

[56] Rooke, T. W., A. T. Hirsch, et al. (2012). "2011 ACCF/AHA focused update of the guideline for the management of patients with peripheral artery disease (updating the 2005 guideline): a report of the American College of Cardiology Foundation/ American Heart Association Task Force on Practice Guidelines: developed in collaboration with the Society for Cardiovascular Angiography and Interventions, Society of Interventional Radiology, Society for Vascular Medicine, and Society for Vascular Surgery." *Catheter Cardiovasc Interv* 79(4): 501-531.

[57] Sacco, R. L., H. C. Diener, et al. (2008). "Aspirin and extended-release dipyridamole versus clopidogrel for recurrent stroke." *N Engl J Med* 359(12): 1238-1251.

[58] Salasidis, G. C., D. A. Latter, et al. (1995). "Carotid artery duplex scanning in preoperative assessment for coronary artery revascularization: the association between peripheral vascular disease, carotid artery stenosis, and stroke." *J Vasc Surg* 21(1): 154-160; discussion 161-152.

[59] Schwartz, L. B., A. H. Bridgman, et al. (1995). "Asymptomatic carotid artery stenosis and stroke in patients undergoing cardiopulmonary bypass." *J Vasc Surg* 21(1): 146-153.

[60] Shahar, E., L. E. Chambless, et al. (2003). "Plasma lipid profile and incident ischemic stroke: the Atherosclerosis Risk in Communities (ARIC) study." *Stroke* 34(3): 623-631.

[61] Shirani, S., M. A. Boroumand, et al. (2006). "Preoperative carotid artery screening in patients undergoing coronary artery bypass graft surgery." *Arch Med Res* 37(8): 987-990.

[62] Tarakji, K. G., J. F. Sabik, 3rd, et al. (2011). "Temporal onset, risk factors, and outcomes associated with stroke after coronary artery bypass grafting." *JAMA* 305(4): 381-390.

[63] Tell, G. S., G. H. Rutan, et al. (1994). "Correlates of blood pressure in community-dwelling older adults. The Cardiovascular Health Study. Cardiovascular Health Study (CHS) Collaborative Research Group." *Hypertension* 23(1): 59-67.

[64] Timaran, C. H., E. B. Rosero, et al. (2008). "Trends and outcomes of concurrent caro-
       tid revascularization and coronary bypass." *J Vasc Surg* 48(2): 355-360; discussion
       360-351.

[65] Van der Heyden, J., M. J. Suttorp, et al. (2007). "Staged carotid angioplasty and stent-
       ing followed by cardiac surgery in patients with severe asymptomatic carotid artery
       stenosis: early and long-term results." *Circulation* 116(18): 2036-2042.

[66] van der Meer, I. M., A. Iglesias del Sol, et al. (2003). "Risk factors for progression of
       atherosclerosis measured at multiple sites in the arterial tree: the Rotterdam Study."
       Stroke 34(10): 2374-2379.

[67] Venkatachalam, S. and M. H. Shishehbor (2011). "Management of carotid disease in
       patients undergoing coronary artery bypass surgery: is it time to change our ap-
       proach?" *Curr Opin Cardiol* 26(6): 480-487.

[68] Versaci, F., B. Reimers, et al. (2009). "Simultaneous hybrid revascularization by caro-
       tid stenting and coronary artery bypass grafting: the SHARP study." *JACC Cardiovasc
       Interv* 2(5): 393-401.

[69] Wilson, P. W., J. M. Hoeg, et al. (1997). "Cumulative effects of high cholesterol levels,
       high blood pressure, and cigarette smoking on carotid stenosis." *N Engl J Med* 337(8):
       516-522.

[70] Yadav, J. S., M. H. Wholey, et al. (2004). "Protected carotid-artery stenting versus en-
       darterectomy in high-risk patients." *N Engl J Med* 351(15): 1493-1501.

[71] Ziada, K. M., J. S. Yadav, et al. (2005). "Comparison of results of carotid stenting fol-
       lowed by open heart surgery versus combined carotid endarterectomy and open
       heart surgery (coronary bypass with or without another procedure)." *Am J Cardiol*
       96(4): 519-523.

Chapter 6

Endovascular Treatment of Ascending Aorta: The Last Frontier?

Eduardo Keller Saadi, Rui Almeida and
Alexandre do Canto Zago

Additional information is available at the end of the chapter

1. Introduction

The treatment of ascending aorta diseases is usually performed by traditional surgery with median sternotomy and cardiopulmonary bypass. However, in some patients, the operative risk of this approach may be prohibitive. In these instances, endovascular approaches to the ascending aorta may be an alternative.

Endovascular approaches are being increasingly utilized to treat a variety of thoracic aortic diseases including aneurysms, pseudoaneurysms, dissections, penetrating aortic ulcers, traumatic aortic rupture, coarctation and abdominal aortic aneurysms [1].

Ascending aorta has several limitations for the endovascular approach, such as its larger diameter and the presence of the aortic valve and the coronary arteries.

2. Access and technique

The endovascular procedure is usually performed through the femoral arteries [1-3]. Sometimes this access is impossible or not recommended because of small size vessels, obstruction, calcification, dissection or extreme tortuosity.

The feasibility of endovascular treatment depends on many anatomic factors, including the diameter and the disease state of the access vessels [4,5]. Stenosis, calcifications, tortuosity, small size or dissection in both femoral and iliac arteries can make introduction of large sheath hazardous or impossible.

Endoprosthesis deployment in the ascending aorta usually requires large diameter and long sheath. There is always possibility of damaging the aortic valve, since the nose of the commercially available devices is designed for descending and/or abdominal aorta. The vascular prosthesis should be large enough to oversize by 15-20 % the aortic diameter and short in length to fit between the coronary arteries and the brachiocephalic trunk. This length usually measures 8 cm or less. The endovascular technique would have several advantages over the open surgical alternatives if the right tools for the procedure were available. Current thoracic aortic stent-grafts are too long, while abdominal aortic stent-grafts are too short and narrow. Moreover, abdominal aortic delivery systems are too short to traverse the long and tortuous path from the femoral artery to the ascending aorta.

Several different approaches have been presented and published over the last years as an attempt to solve very dramatic situations stretching the limits of the current technology [6-8].

The technique should be carefully planned. Rapid pacing and adenosine are useful to lower blood pressure and allow precise deployment. A rigid (Landerquist or super stiff) and long (260 cm) guidewire is usually placed in the left ventricle to give adequate support near the coronary arteries. This is similar to what we use when performing transcatheter aortic valve implantation (TAVI). One important tip is to perform a "wide J-shape" at the end of the rigid guidewire in order to prevent left ventricule perforation and, consequently, cardiac tamponade or left ventricular pseudoaneurysm.

Similar to other endovascular procedures, besides careful planning, patient selection and technical expertise are crucial to obtain satisfactory results. In this setting multidetector computed tomography (MDCT) plays an important role in selecting the patients suitable for the procedure and allows a careful and detailed step by step preoperative planning.

We have recently published a series of five clinical cases and described the technique in which the axillary artery was used to deliver the endograft for the treatment of different thoracic aortic diseases [9]. We also demonstrated the possibility of concomitant treatment of ascending aorta disease and coronary stent implantation [10,11].

Transcarotid is another alternative access and, recently, transapical approach through a small left thoracotomy has been described.

3. Clinical cases

In this part we will discuss clinical cases of endovascular treatment of ascending aortic diseases showing different approaches and techniques.

3.1. Clinical case 1

A 32-year-old female presenting cardiogenic shock (Figures 1-2).

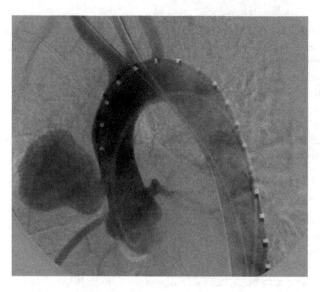

Figure 1. Aortogram showing bovine trunk and a pseudoaneurysm in the anterolateral wall of the ascending aorta 1 cm above the ostium of the right coronary artery.

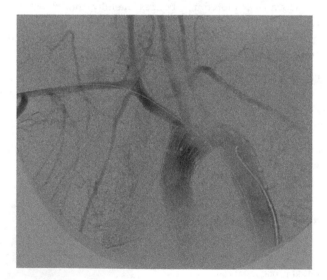

Figure 2. Final aortogram of emergency endovascular correction of a pseudoaneurysm through transfemoral implantation of a Cook endoprosthesis. The shorter device we had available was a 8 cm length endoprosthesis. In order to preserve flow in the brachiocephalic trunk and left carotid artery (bovine trunk) we had to use a chimney (snorkel) technique in this two vessels arch using two Viabahns to preserve flow.

3.2. Clinical case 2

A 57-year-old female underwent coronary artery bypass graft in another hospital with left internal mammary artery to the left anterior descending and saphenous vein graft to the right coronary artery. The patient developed mediastinitis and had 7 reinterventions resulting in acute bleeding through the sternum. She was sent to our hospital in cardiogenic shock and manual compression of the bleeding site in the sternum. Previous computed tomography showed ruptured pseudoaneurysm at the proximal anastomosis of saphenous vein graft to the (Figures 3-6).

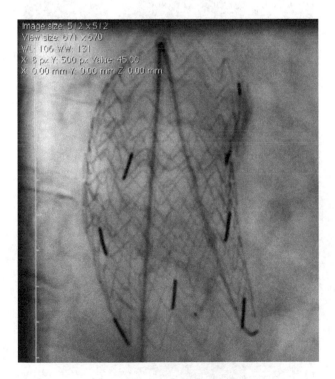

Figure 3. Emergency endovascular deployment of two abdominal extension cuffs (Gore-Tex) in the ascending aorta between the coronary ostium and the brachiocephalic trunk through the left axillary artery. The bleeding stopped immediately and the patient became stable.

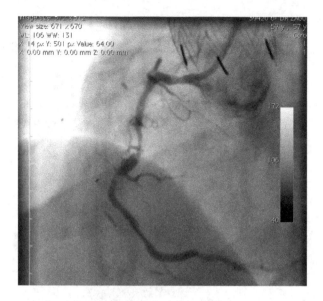

Figure 4. Right coronary angiography demonstrating severe stenosis. Once saphenous vein graft to the right coronary artery had occluded by the endoprosthesis, the native right coronary artery had to be treated.

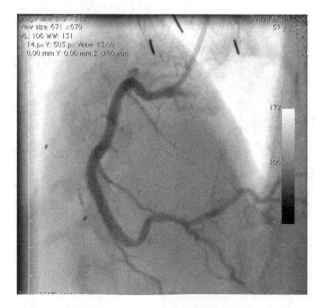

Figure 5. Deployment of three stents in the right coronary artery.

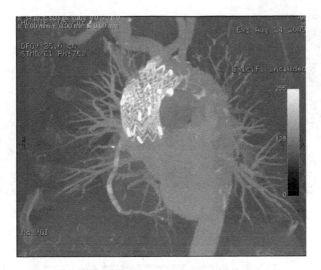

Figure 6. Computed tomography showing the two extension cuffs in the ascending aorta and the three stents in the right coronary artery.

3.3. Clinical case 3

A 74-year-old male with previous coronary artery bypass graft presented with iatrogenic ascending aortic pseudoaneurysm that occurred during angiography. The patient was at very high risk for surgical treatment, therefore an (Figures 7-9).

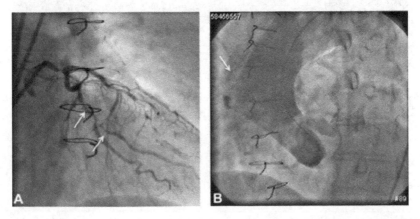

Figure 7. A) Coronary angiogram showing left main bifurcation with severe stenosis and circumflex with severe stenosis extending to large marginal branch. (B) Aortic angiogram demonstrating ascending aorta dilatation and image suggesting dissection at the saphenous vein graft ostium.

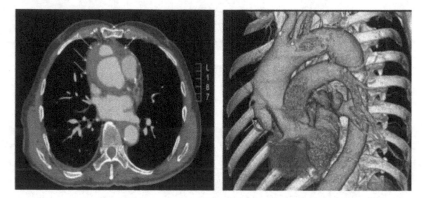

Figure 8. Computerized tomographic angiography showing a 3.4-cm pseudoaneurysm with partial thrombosis in ascending aorta and surrounding intramural hematoma.

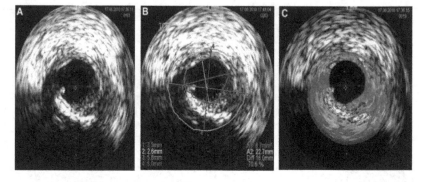

Figure 9. A) Intravascular ultrasound of left main artery evidencing significant stenosis due to calcified plaque. (B) Intravascular ultrasound measurements confirming the presence of a large left main artery and significant plaque burden. (C) Virtual histology showing predominantly fibrous plaque and superficial calcium arch.

Both procedures were successfully performed and the patient was discharged without (Figures 10-12). At 6 months and 1 year clinical follow-up the patient had no symptoms as well as no other adverse cardiovascular events.

4. Target diseases

There are several pathologies of the ascending aorta that can be potentially addressed by the endovascular approach. Pseudoaneurysms or sacular aneurysms in the mid-ascending aorta are adequate for this technique because they usually appear with a sufficient proximal and

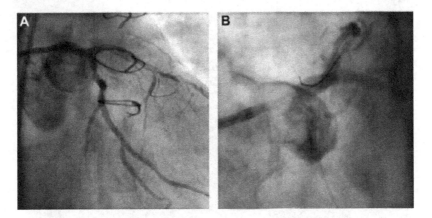

Figure 10. Coronary angiogram showing final result in right anterior oblique projection (A) and spider view (B).

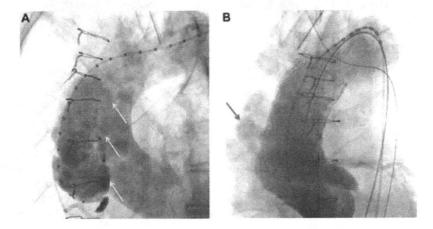

Figure 11. (A) Ascending aorta angiogram before endoprosthesis deployment showing a large pseudoaneurysm (yellow arrow). (B) Ascending aorta angiogram after endoprosthesis deployment evidencing sealed pseudoaneurysm and a type 1 endoleak (red arrow).

distal landing zone. On the other hand, fusiform aneurysms have the limitation of lacking a sufficient landing zone in many cases.

Thoracic endovascular stent grafting has revolutionized the treatment of distal [type B] acute aortic dissection. Endovascular surgeons are now seeking the ways to improve the treatment of type A dissection by offering endovascular techniques to replace conventional surgical therapy. Less invasive endovascular therapy, obviates the need for sternotomy and cardiopulmonary bypass, reduces perioperative morbidity, and offers an alternative solution for

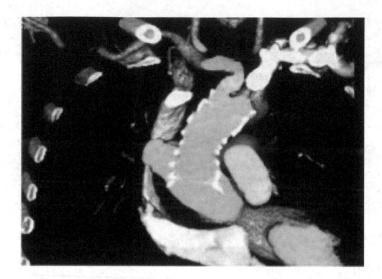

Figure 12. Computerized tomographic angiography showing final result after endoprosthesis deployment.

those patients not eligible for conventional intervention due to co-morbidity or severe complications of the disease.

Thoracic stent grafting in the ascending aorta presents specific challenges and the role of uncovered stents is unclear in this situation. The majority of patients with acute type A aortic dissection has the intimal tear originated in the sinotubular junction. More than 90% of patients with this disease does not have sufficient proximal or distal landing zone required for secure fixation. Therefore, the site of the intimal tear as well as aortic valve insufficiency and aortic diameter >38mm are major factors limiting the use of endovascular therapy for acute type A dissection. Current available stents in use to treat type B aortic dissection do not address anatomical constraints present in type A aortic dissection in the majority of cases, hence the development of new devices is required.

5. Technical limitations

Endovascular approach of the ascending aorta has several limitations and is still in its beginning phase.

The diameter of the ascending aorta is usually larger than the rest of the aorta and the proximity with the aortic valve and the presence of the coronary arteries pose special challenges.

The length of the delivery system, which is designed for the abdominal aorta, does not allow to reach the ascending aorta through the groin.

Finally, the length of the endoprosthesis itself for descending aorta may be too long to be positioned between the coronary ostia and the brachiocephalic trunk.

6. Conclusions

Despite the fantastic progress in this field and the clear advantages of endovascular approaches for the ascending aorta in some clinical situations, one must bear in mind the high level of risk that these procedures entail.

Long-term data are not available to establish the safety and durability of stent-graft repairs. The cases described represent an off-label use of this technology and should be considered with the above mentioned limitations in mind.

The surgeon will need special skills in open aortic surgery and catheter based interventions to be able to plan the procedure carefully, to properly deliver the devices and to manage the potential serious complications [12].

Challenges in endograft design are the development of branched endografts and of pathology-specific endografts [13]. However, the unique composition of the proximal thoracic aorta and the associated mechanical properties have to be taken into account and make this effort by far more complex than initially expected. Moreover, there is a need for reducing the stent-graft devices profile as well as for increasing conformability and trackability.

We believe that future advances with devices specifically designed for the treatment of ascending aorta diseases will allow this technique to be incorporated into routine medical practice.

Author details

Eduardo Keller Saadi[1,2,3], Rui Almeida[4,5,6] and Alexandre do Canto Zago[1,2,7]

1 Federal University of Rio Grande do Sul, Porto Alegre, RS, Brazil

2 Federal University of Rio Grande do Sul Hospital, Porto Alegre, RS, Brazil

3 Mãe de Deus Hospital, Porto Alegre, RS, Brazil

4 West Paraná State University, Cascavel, PR, Brazil

5 Mãe de Deus Hospital, Cascavel, PR, Brazil

6 Cardiovascular Surgery Institute of West Paraná, Cascavel, PR, Brazil

7 Lutheran University Hospital, Porto Alegre, RS, Brazil

References

[1] Melissano, G, Bertoglio, L, Civilini, E, Marone, E. M, Calori, G, Setacci, F, & Chiesa, R. Results of Thoracic Endovascular Grafting in Different Aortic Segments. J Endovasc Ther (2007). , 14, 150-157.

[2] Guidelines for the Diagnosis and Management of Patients with Thoracic Aortic DiseaseA Report of the American College of Cardiology Foundation/American Heart Association Task Force on Practice Guidelines, American Association for Thoracic Surgery, American College of Radiology, American Stroke Association, Society of Cardiovascular Anesthesiologists, Society for Cardiovascular Angiography and Interventions, Society of Interventional Radiology, Society of Thoracic Surgeons, and Society for Vascular Medicine. Circulation (2010). ee369., 266.

[3] Nienaber, C. A, Rousseau, H, Eggebrecht, H, Kische, S, Fattori, R, Rehders, T. C, Kundt, G, Scheinert, D, Czerny, M, Kleinfeldt, T, Zipfel, B, & Labrousse, L. Ince HS for the INSTEAD Trial. Randomized Comparison of Strategies for Type B Aortic Dissection. Circulation (2009). , 120, 2519-2528.

[4] Alric, P, Canaud, L, Branchereau, P, Marty-ané, C, & Berthet, J. P. Preoperative assessment of anatomical suitability for thoracic endovascular aortic repair. Acta Chir Belg (2009). , 109(4), 458-64.

[5] Almeida, R. M, Leal, J. C, Saadi, E. K, & Braile, D. M. Rocha AST, Volpiani J, Centola C, Zago A. Thoracic endovascular aortic repair- a Brazilian experience in 255 patients over a period of 112 months. Interact CardioVasc Thorac Surg (2009). , 524-528.

[6] Uchida, K, Imoto, K, Yanagi, H, Machida, D, Okiyama, M, Yasuda, S, et al. Endovascular Repair of Ascending Aortic Rupture: Effectiveness of a Fenestrated Stent-Graft. J Endovasc Ther (2010). , 17, 395-398.

[7] Lin, P, Kougias, P, Huynh, T, Huh, J, & Coselli, J. S. Endovascular Repair of Ascending Aortic Pseudoaneurysm: Technical Considerations of a Common Carotid Artery Approach Using the Zenith Aortic Cuff Endograft. J Endovasc Ther (2007).

[8] Chuter TAMEndovascular Repair in the Ascending Aorta: Stretching the Limits of Current Technology. J Endovasc Ther (2007). , 14, 799-800.

[9] Saadi, E. K, Dussin, L. H, Moura, L, & Machado, A. S. The axillary artery--a new approach for endovascular treatment of thoracic aortic diseases. Interact Cardiovasc Thorac Surg. (2010). Nov;, 11(5), 617-9.

[10] Zago, A. C, Saadi, E. K, & Zago, A. J. Endovascular approach to treat ascending aortic pseudoaneurysm in a patient with previous CABG and very high surgical risk. Catheter Cardiovasc Interv. (2011). Oct 1;, 78(4), 551-7.

[11] Saadi, E. K. Moura Ld, Zago A, Zago A. Endovascular repair of ascending aorta and coronary stent implantation.Rev Bras Cir Cardiovasc. (2011). Jul-Sep;, 26(3), 477-80.

[12] Saadi, E. K. Is it possible to train an endovascular surgeon? Rev Bras Cir Cardiovasc. (2007). Jan-Mar;22(1):III-IV.

[13] Greenberg, R, Eagleton, M, & Mastracci, T. Branched endografts for thoracoabdominal aneurysms. J Thorac Cardiovasc Surg (2010). S, 171-8.

Chapter 7

Impact of Renal Dysfunction and Peripheral Arterial Disease on Post-Operative Outcomes After Coronary Artery Bypass Grafting

Muhammad A. Chaudhry, Zainab Omar and
Faisal Latif

Additional information is available at the end of the chapter

1. Introduction

In-hospital and long-term outcomes after Coronary artery Bypass grafting (CABG) are impacted by various factors including age, gender and various co-morbidities including chronic obstructive pulmonary disease, hypertension, diabetes Mellitus, dyslipidemia, chronic kidney disease (CKD), Peripheral arterial disease (PAD) and even connective tissue disorders such as systemic lupus erythematosus, and rheumatoid arthritis.

Both CKD and PAD have been considered a major risk factor for morbidity and mortality post-CABG [1]. Therefore, both are always considered as a variable when calculating risk for perioperative mortality in patients undergoing CABG in the popular EUROSCORE and society of Society of Thoracic Surgeons National Cardiac Surgery Database scoring system [1,2].

We will discuss the degree of importance of these co-morbidities along with the epidemiology, underlying proposed pathogenetic mechanisms, significant associated co-factors, and also highlight the pertinent existing data on these parameters.

2. CKD and its impact on outcomes after CABG

Chronic kidney disease is defined as derangement in renal function for a period of at least six months. It is broadly divided into five stages based on creatinine clearance or glomerular filtration rate (GFR) obtained from either Cockcroft-Gault or modification of diet in renal disease (MDRD) equations [3,4]:

Cockcroft-Gault equation: Creatinine Clearance (ml/min) = [([140 − age] × weight [kg])/72 × serum creatinine (mg/dl)] (× 0.85 for women),

MDRD equation: GFR (mL/min/1.73 m^2) = 175 × (serum creatinine)$^{-1.154}$ × (Age)$^{-0.203}$ × (0.742 if female) × (1.212 if African American) (conventional units)

Creatinine clearance or glomerular filtration rate (GFR) represents renal function. Declining values represent a decline in renal function. Stage 1 refers to glomerular filtration rate (GFR) >90 ml/min and is generally asymptomatic. GFR between 60-90 ml/min is stage 2 CKD. Stage 3 is GFR between 30 and 60 ml/min and is further subdivided into Stage 3A (GFR 45-60 ml/min) and Stage 3B (GFR 30-45 ml/min). Stage 4 is defined by GFR between 15-30 ml/min while GFR <15 ml/min signifies Stage 5 and is considered an indication for renal replacement therapy i.e. dialysis. The most common etiological factors for CKD include diabetes mellitus and hypertension resulting in diabetic nephropathy and hypertensive nephrosclerosis, respectively.

The presence of CKD is considered a major independent predictor for development of coronary artery disease (CAD). An analysis from the atherosclerosis risk in communities (ARIC) study, Manjunath et al demonstrated that in 15,350 subjects with a mean follow up of over 6 years, there was a significant increase in acute coronary syndrome events in patients with stage 3 and 4 CKD (14.2%) compared with 5.5% in patients with stage 1 CKD (HR 1.38 (1.02, 1.87). Additionally, with every 10 ml/min/1.73 m^2 decline in GFR, there was a progressive increase in the incidence of cardiac events [5].

2.1. Proposed pathogenic mechanisms

Many factors contribute in the mechanisms associated in the renal contribution to increased risk of cardiovascular events. We briefly discuss a few here: Impaired renal function is associated with reduced erythropoietin synthesis and consequent anemia, which has been associated with cardiovascular disease [6]. Reduced 1, 25 (OH) vitamin D synthesis is associated with increased parathyroid hormone levels and higher prevalence of vascular calcification and arteriosclerosis [7].

Abnormal calcium phosphate metabolism is a consequence of renal dysfunction and it has a strong association with increased adverse cardiovascular events. Hyperphosphatemia and hypercalcemia are distinctly independent risk factors leading to a greater occurrence of cardiovascular events in patients with CKD and additionally, are also associated with poor surgical outcomes in patients undergoing CABG. Increased calcium-phosphate product greater than 55 and hyperphosphatemia escalates the development of secondary hyperparathyroidism which has been linked to increased osteoclastic activity and enhanced calcium-phosphate precipitation in the vasculature. There is also increase in the number of protein receptors in vessel cell membrane which increases deposition of calcium. In patients with CKD, vitamin D deficiency is also present even in the early stages. Vitamin D levels have a pivotal role in calcium-phosphorus homeostasis, regulation of parathyroid hormone (PTH), and bone metabolism and turnover. Three plausible mechanisms have been suggested in the protective effects of vitamin D against cardiovascular disease mortality are that vitamin D can inhibit various foci of inflammation which is a key pathogenic mechanism in atherosclerosis; vitamin D also has an anti-proliferative effect on myocardial cell hypertrophy and proliferation and prevents remodeling which underlies the pathogenesis of congestive heart failure and vitamin D acts as an inhibitory endocrine regulator for the renin-angiotensin system, which triggers the cascade of hypertension and decompensated heart failure[8]. Thus, with low 1,25 hydroxy cholecalciferol levels, this effect is pronounced causing even further increase in cardiovascular risk.

We will discuss the outcomes of patients with CKD with the two modes of revascularization namely percutaneous and then, surgical. Additionally, we will take into account the impact of various comorbidities such as diabetes, dyslipidemias with respect to lipoprotein levels as well as the role of oxidative stress in this patient population.

Although long-term mortality may improve with surgical revascularization in dialysis patients with coronary artery disease, perioperative mortality continues to remain higher among patients with end-stage renal disease (ESRD) requiring CABG. Various studies have compared the outcomes of percutaneous coronary intervention (PCI) versus CABG and showed that mortality is not different [9-11]. However, these studies were from the 1990s and percutaneous techniques have been refined since then with improved outcomes. Newer studies are required to compare outcomes of percutaneous versus surgical revascularization.

2.2. Outcomes with percutaneous coronary intervention

In hemodialysis dependent patients (CKD stage 5), clinical outcomes of PCI are especially poor. Before the advent of coronary stents 20 years ago, when percutaneous revascularization was performed with balloon angioplasty alone, it was found that patients with ESRD experience a higher rate of coronary restenosis and recurrent angina, when compared to patients without ESRD [12]. In another case control study of twenty patients with ESRD and 20 age and sex matched controls without renal disease, it was shown that the rate of restenosis was 60% in ESRD patients, as compared to 35% in patients without renal disease. Restenosis was found to be dependent on size of vessel dilated and there was increased prothrombotic risk secondary to increased fibrinogen concentrations [13].

Many patients with ESRD experience silent ischemia. The possible mechanism being uremic polyneuropathy and therefore, may not experience typical ischemic symptoms.

In a prospective study of 5327 patients undergoing percutaneous coronary intervention (PCI) with a follow up of over five years, rate of death or myocardial infarction at one year was 1.5% in CKD patients with creatinine clearance >70 ml/min, 3.6% in patients with creatinine clearance between 50-70 ml/min, 7.8% between 30 and 49 ml/min and 18.1% with creatinine clearance less than 30ml/min. This study showed a progressive increase in adverse outcomes with worsening renal function. CKD was a strong predictor of adverse cardiovascular events including death and MI [14].

2.3. CABG in patients with renal dysfunction

Even though conflicting studies exist, a large study has shown that although there is increased risk of mortality in patients with ESRD undergoing CABG when compared to patients without significant renal disease, it still portends a better outcome in terms of mortality when compared to percutaneous revascularization in this patient population [15].

2.4. Hard endpoints after CABG

It has been shown that the lower the GFR, the worse the mortality after CABG. In a study of 2067 patients, it was found that estimated GFR was a powerful and independent predictor of mortality in multivariate analysis. Estimated average GFR in patients who died was 57.9+/-17.6 mL/min per 1.73 m^2 mg/dl, as compared to 64.7 +/- 13.8 mL/min per 1.73 m^2 in those who survived at an average follow-up for 2.3 years [16].

In a database review of 483,914 CABG patients over a three year period, it was shown that the post-operative mortality rates for stage 2, stage 3, and stage 4 CKD patients were 1.8%, 4.3% and 9.3 % respectively. Also, there was a higher incidence of stroke, need for re-operation, sternal infection, prolonged mechanical ventilation greater than 48 hours and a hospital stay of longer than two weeks [17]. In a prospective study of 15,500 CABG patients over a five year period, it was shown that dialysis dependent patients with CABG had higher risk of in-hospital mortality as compared to non- dialysis dependent CABG patients (12.2% as compared to 3.1%) and also significantly higher risk of mediastinitis (3.6 vs. 1.2%) [18].

One of the largest initial studies on CABG outcomes in ESRD patients 13 years ago was a retrospective study on 82 patients in which patients had a mean follow-up of 3 years. 18.5 % of the patients had left ventricular ejection fraction (LVEF) <0.45 and the aortic cross clamp time was fairly good at 50 ± 3 minutes [10]. Mean number of grafts was 2.3. Sixty-two percent of patients received left internal mammary grafts. In this study, 30-day mortality rate was 14.6%, and the mean survival rate at one, three and five years was 71%, 56% and 39% respectively. Thirty day mortality was 14.6% due to a variety of causes including myocardial infarction, cardiac arrest or cardiac tamponade. This study showed that although there was high peri and post- operative as well as long term mortality in ESRD patients undergoing CABG, there was a significant improvement in functional status as a result of CABG. The use of internal mammary artery grafts was related with less in-hospital mortality as well. Perioperative atrial fibrillation occurred in 12.1 % of patients within the first thirty days. With patients having preoperative Newyork Heart Association (NYHA) class III or class IV symptoms, LVEF less than 45% and age greater than 60 years, there was higher long term mortality. The incidence of post- operative bleeding and sternal infection was 3.6% which was higher when compared to patients not on dialysis.

Patients with CKD have a poor baroreceptor reflex. Therefore, they do not adjust very well in conditions like post-operative hypotension. Therefore, poor cardiac output can be more symptomatic in this group of patients [19].

In a study of 2438 CKD patients undergoing CABG over a three year period, operative mortality was 4.8% in individuals with stage 3 CKD and 7.1% in individuals with stage 4–5 CKD while it was 2.2% in those without significant CKD [20]. CKD was associated with increased post-operative blood transfusion requirement, acute kidney injury superimposed on CKD, myocardial injury and cardiac arrest. Use of blood transfusions and acute kidney injury were strongly associated with in-hospital death in CKD patients.

2.5. Impact of mode of dialysis on outcomes after CABG

The mode of dialysis is equally important in influencing CABG outcomes, namely perito-neal (PD) and hemo-dialysis (HD). Peritoneal dialysis has been associated with worse out-comes when compared with hemodialysis [21,22]. Following CABG, diaphragmatic splinting, atelectasis and hypoxemia can occur after early post-operative initiation of PD. In a retrospective analysis of 105 patients, among whom 40 were on PD, and 65 on HD and all patients had been on dialysis for at least 2 months prior to CABG, it was demonstrated that the incidence of post- operative dialysate leak and peritonitis was 10% and 12.5% respective-ly in patients on PD. On the other hand, incidence of arterio-venous access thrombosis was 4.6% in patients on HD. Besides older age, PD was an independent risk factor of high opera-tive mortality (adjusted OR for in hospital mortality in PD patients was 22.58). Actual causes of mortality included sepsis, cardiac arrest, pneumonia and gastrointestinal bleed. Chief in-fective organisms in septic patients were Staphylococcus aureus (coagulase negative), Pseu-domonas aeruginosa, and Enterococcus faecalis [21]. Risk of peritonitis is higher if gastroepiploic artery is harvested for CABG as it requires diaphragmatic incision [22].

2.6. Impact of comorbidities in patients with CKD undergoing CABG

Diabetes and hypertension are the most common causes of CKD and they are also the major risk factors for coronary artery disease, therefore, the incidence of CAD is higher in these patients.

2.6.1. Diabetes

Diabetes is present in almost one third of CKD patients undergoing CABG and is considered a strong predictor of mortality in this patient group [23,24].

Szabo et al showed in a study of 2779 CABG patients that in 19.4% of patients with diabetes, the cross-clamp and cardiopulmonary bypass times as well as the need for inotropic sup-port, transfusion of blood products and progression of renal failure were all higher in pa-tients with CKD. Additionally, the incidence of post-operative stroke was greater in diabetic patients (4.3% vs. 1.7%). Five year survival rate was 84.4% in diabetic group while it was 91.3% in the non- diabetic group [25]. Another study showed that diabetes was an inde-pendent major predictor of morbidity and mortality in CABG patients. In 12,198 patients, it was observed that the diabetic group had higher rates of post-operative mortality (3.9% vs. 1.6%) and stroke (2.9% vs. 1.4%). The five and ten year survival rates were 78% and 50% among patients with diabetes as compared to 88 and 71% in the non-diabetic group [26]. Morris et al demonstrated in a study of 5654 patients undergoing CABG that the five year survival rate for diabetic patients was 80% as compared to 91% for non- diabetics [27]. Out-comes of CABG are improved in diabetic patients who undergo grafting of internal mam-mary arteries, with two being better than one. In a retrospective analysis of 4382 patients undergoing CABG, it was shown at 10 year follow-up that bilateral internal mammary artery grafting in addition to SVGs in diabetic patients improved survival and decreased need for revascularization compared with single internal mammary artery grafting along with SVGs [28]. The strong correlation between diabetes and cardiovascular outcomes including survival and myocardial infarction is due to the diffusely extensive and rapidly progressive nature of atherosclerotic coronary artery disease (CAD) in this group of patients. Various other factors such as oxidized low-density lipoproteins (LDL), hyperglycemia causing adverse metabolic shifts, deranged fibrinolysis, increased coagulability, and advanced renovascular hypertension resulting in change in vessel architecture also contribute to the progressive nature of CAD in diabetics. There is increased tendency for LDL induced atherosclerotic plaque formation and there is greater predisposition to thrombosis due to increased blood viscosity secondary to high plasma protein levels. There is also platelet and endothelial dysfunction and increased production of thromboxane A2 and von- willebrand factor along with decreased production of prostacyclins which creates a procoagulant state. Coronary vasodilation is impaired as a result of loss of the hyperpolarizing mechanics normally present in endothelial cells. Autonomic neuropathy in diabetes increases cardiac chrontropic workload and subsequently leads to greater oxygen demand even at rest. There is enhanced vascular tone in the coronary atherosclerotic plaque area leading to further reduction in blood flow, producing orthostatic changes which leads to reduction in coronary perfusion pressure and mitigates warning signs of ischemia such as angina [27,29-32].

2.6.2. Hypertension

Hypertension has also been associated with worse post CABG outcomes. In a multi centre study of 2417 patients among whom patients were categorized into patients with normal preoperative blood pressure, isolated systolic hypertension (systolic blood pressure >140 mm Hg), diastolic hypertension (diastolic blood pressure >90 mm Hg), or a combination of systolic and diastolic hypertension. It was found that isolated systolic hypertension was associated with a 40% greater risk of adverse outcomes such as stroke, renal failure, congestive heart failure and all cause mortality after CABG. Even after correction for confounding risk factor adjustment, the increased risk of adverse outcomes was significantly more pronounced in hypertensive patients [33].

2.6.3. Impact of other risk factors

In a study of 936 hemodialysis patients to elucidate correlation of recognized risk factors in CKD patients, it was found that correlation with diabetes, smoking, African-American race and increasing age of above fifty- five years was strong. It is suspected that non-traditional risk factors like uremic environment and hemodialysis procedure using arteriovenous fistulae and high output state associated with these fistulae also impact the outcomes after CABG adversely [34].

Dyslipidemia with a high LDL is a classic risk factor for development of CAD in the general population. However, it is likely not a major risk factor in patients with advanced renal disease. In a study of 210 dialysis dependent patients compared with 223 control subjects with normal renal function, it was found that high density lipoprotein (HDL) levels were low while intermediate and very low density lipoprotein (IDL and VLDL) levels as well as tri-glyceride levels were higher in dialysis patients while there was no significant difference in LDL levels [35]. In part, the role of decreased renal metabolism of lipids leads to a decreased level of LDL is likely the cause.

Atherosclerosis is regarded as an inflammatory process [36]. It has also been shown that in dialysis-dependent patients, oxidative stress is increased resulting in a pro-inflammatory en-vironment. As a result, incidence of cardiovascular events is increased. In a comparison study of 28 healthy subjects and 31 patients with renal disease, it was discovered that gluta-thione peroxidase and superoxide dismutase activities were increased in patients on HD while total glutathione and glutathione reductase activity is reduced resulting in increased oxidative stress [37].

2.6.4. Impact of renal artery stenosis on CABG

Renal artery stenosis (RAS) can lead to refractory hypertension and gradual deterioration in kidney function. The presence of underlying RAS and its effect on CABG outcomes has been studied and variable results have been obtained. In a study of 798 patients undergoing iso-lated CABG with 18.7% having renal artery stenosis (>50% stenosis), acute renal failure de-veloped in 10.2% of patients post procedure. The mortality rate was 14% in patients who developed acute renal failure (ARF) post operatively, while it was 0.2% in patients who did not develop ARF. However, presence of RAS was not associated with development of ARF post-operatively [38].

In a series of eighteen patients undergoing CABG who also had varying degrees of RAS with mean serum creatinine of 2.6±2.7 mg/dl, RAS was not associated with adverse out-comes post-operatively [39].

2.7. Post-CABG complications in patients with CKD

Besides relatively increased short-term mortality in patients with CKD undergoing CABG, they also encounter increased morbidity from infections, blood transfusions, and stroke. In a retrospective analysis of 3954 patients where 82.7% patients had creatinine <1.5 mg/dl, and 16% had a serum creatinine level between 1.5 and 3.0 mg/dl, it was demonstrated that pa-tients with a serum creatinine level >1.5 mg/dl had a mortality of 7% compared to 3% in pa-tients with serum creatinine <1.5 mg/dl. Additionally, patients with a higher serum creatinine level had a higher incidence of requiring prolonged mechanical ventilation (15% vs. 8%), risk of stroke (7% vs. 2%), and bleeding complications (8% vs. 3%). Three infectious complications (mediastinitis, graft harvest site infection, and chest wound infections) were not different among these groups, whereas the occurrence of pneumonia and endocarditis was significantly higher in patients with a higher serum creatinine [40].

2.7.1. Prolonged mechanical ventilation

It is believed that the prolonged mechanical ventilation and the need for re-intubation after CABG in patients with renal dysfunction are due to a compromised ability to eliminate fluid volume, thereby predisposing patients to impaired alveolar gas exchange. Additionally, renal failure would result in decreased metabolism and elimination of sedative, anxiolytic and analgesic drugs leading to impairment of respiratory drive.

A study showed that ventilatory complications such as need for greater than 48 hours of mechanical ventilation and re- intubation is high in patients with significant renal dysfunction undergoing CABG, when compared to patients with normal or mild renal dysfunction [40]. Another study showed a stepwise increase in need for prolonged mechanical ventilation as the renal function deteriorates. In this study, the ventilator dependence rate greater than 24 hours was 8.6%, 14.7%, and 20.2%, as the stage of CKD increased [20].

2.7.2. Bleeding complications post CABG

Platelet dysfunction is a consequence of uremia in patients with CKD and they are more prone to bleeding complications requiring blood transfusion. A study showed that significant renal dysfunction (serum creatinine of 1.5 to 3.0 mg/dl) significantly increases bleeding complications such as disseminated intravascular coagulation, gastrointestinal hemorrhage, or thoracic hemorrhage sufficient to require reoperation, or result in cardiac complications such as cardiac arrest and low cardiac output [40].

The association of transfusion with mortality is particularly interesting. CKD impairs erythropoiesis in the bone marrow due to reduced synthesis of erythropoietin, and is associated with pre-operative anemia of chronic disease and also leads to increased risk of bleeding after CABG [41]. Strategies to optimize preoperative hemoglobin and to minimize post-operative transfusion could possibly improve operative outcomes in patients with CKD. Transfusion needs are also increased as a result of uremia induced platelet dysfunction which can cause an increase in bleeding tendency in these patients.

2.7.3. Other post-CABG complications in CKD

Interestingly, occurrence of post-operative atrial fibrillation has been shown to increase with worsening renal function as well. In a study, the occurrence of atrial fibrillation was 22.2%. 19.2% and 16.5% in severe, moderate and mild CKD patients respectively [20].

Different studies have demonstrated the increased incidence of stroke in patients with CKD. In an analysis on 2438 patients undergoing CABG, the incidence of stroke was 3%, 2.7% and 1.7% in severe, moderate and mild CKD groups [20].

Infectious complications occur more commonly in patients with CKD undergoing CABG as well. A study showed that deep sternal infection, pneumonia, septicemia, infection involving a leg vein and overall infection rate was higher as the CKD stage increased (9.0%, 5.1%, and 3.5% in severe, moderate and mild CKD respectively) [20].

2.8. Impact of aortic cross clamp time in CABG

Aortic cross clamping time is the period during which an occlusive clamp is placed on the ascending aorta close to the innominate artery as a part of achieving cardioplegia before proceeding with coronary bypass grafting. The mechanism of induction of cardioplegia involves prevention of repolarization of myocardial cell membrane due to the high potassium concentration of the cardioplegic fluid causing inactivation of the sodium channels which initiate the action potential. The hypothermic fluid of cardioplegia induces asystole. When the solution is administered in the aortic root it is termed antegrade and when administered in the coronary sinus, it is called retrograde. Myocardial protection with cardioplegia decreases the energy demands of the heart by arrest of the contractile apparatus. This is considered to be an extension of ischemia tolerance which is considered to minimize the deleterious effects of induced cardiac arrest. However, it still is desirable to keep duration of cardioplegia at a minimum as the aortic cross-clamp time is an important factor in predicting mortality in cardiac surgery and the lesser it is, the better the outcomes. The metabolic processes resulting from cardiac ischemia include sudden cessation of normal aerobic cardiac metabolic events, reduction in creatine phosphate, initiation of anaerobic glycolysis, and build-up of lactate and alpha glycerol phosphate as well as nucleotide metabolites. This is associated with contractile impairment and electrical pathway alterations consistent with typical EKG changes. The myocardial demand for high energy phosphate substrates is increased when the availability of adenosine triphosphate decreases. The predominant mode of energy derivation is switched to anaerobic glycolysis in the ischemic tissue. With early ischemic component, contractile activity and later on ion transport utilizes available adenosine triphosphate but gradually with the increase in ischemic time period, the metabolic demands undergo a compensatory reduction to prevent further ischemic damage. Irreversible injury in cardiac muscle is highlighted by very low levels of adenosine triphosphate, lack of energy production even by anaerobic mode, progressive accumulation of hydrogen ions, adenosine monophosphate, and lactic acid with a consequently high osmotic load, mitochondrial swelling and amorphous densities in matrix, and loss of integrity of the sarcolemmal membrane. The precise mechanism of pathogenesis is still elusive. In animal models, severe ischemia causes irreversible cell injury and death in one hour while with less severe ischemia in the mid and sub-epicardial myocardium, survival is possible up to six hours. Irreversible injury and cell death after six hours is inevitable. The ischemic injury changes reverse to a certain degree after reperfusion but how quickly and completely this transformation occurs is highly variable ranging from minutes to days. Aerobic metabolism is restored early while adenine nucleotide pool and stunning resolve slowly [42].

Systolic dysfunction with reduction in LVEF <0.40 is also an indicator of poor prognosis in CKD patients undergoing CABG. In a comparison study of aortic cross clamp times in patients with normal versus reduced ejection fraction in 27,215 patients in which 99.8 % received antegrade, retrograde or combined cardioplegia, it was found that prolonged aortic cross clamp time was an independent predictor of mortality [43]. It was shown that a combination of reduced LVEF and prolonged aortic cross clamp time especially with CKD compounds the ischemic effects and increases overall risk of perioperative mortality. In this study, the mean aortic cross clamp time was 68± 20 minutes, number of distal grafts was 3.1± 1.4 and 68.7% of patients underwent grafting of the left internal mammary artery. The incidence of pulmonary complications was 12.2% and stroke was 2.27%. Fifty-two percent of the patients had baseline hypertension, 29% had diabetes and 7% were dialysis dependent.

It has been shown that patients undergoing CABG with off pump or beating heart technique experience improved post-operative outcomes and less perioperative mortality. In a study of 638 patients with acute coronary syndrome undergoing emergency CABG out of which 240 were operated off pump and 398 had standard on-pump CABG. 14.5% of patients were in cardiogenic shock along with serum creatinine greater than 1.8 mg /dl. Follow-up was up to 5 years. The results showed that in the off pump CABG group, in-hospital outcomes were significantly better. With off-pump CABG, skin incision to culprit lesion revascularization time was significantly reduced. There was less requirement for prolonged mechanical venti-lation, less need for inotropic support, less incidence of atrial fibrillation, lower stroke rate (2.5 % vs. 6.7%), shorter intensive care unit stay and less sternal wound healing complica-tions (2.5% vs. 3.5%). The overall hospital mortality rate was also reduced (5.7%) as com-pared to those on cardiopulmonary bypass (8.6%) [44].

2.9. Conclusion

As we have discussed, numerous studies have shown that patients with CKD have worse outcomes including an increased mortality and other complications after undergoing CABG, when compared to patients without CKD. However, an increasing number of patients with ESRD continue to undergo CABG and additionally, these patients are getting more complex a higher presence of comorbidities including diabetes, hypertension and obesity [Figure 1]. However, fortunately, in-hospital mortality rates have declined remarkably from over 31% to 5.4% in patients with ESRD (versus 4.7% to 1.8% among patients without ESRD) [45]. However, the mortality in ESRD patients remains 3-fold higher which indicates the need of continued work to improve outcomes in these patients [Figure 2].

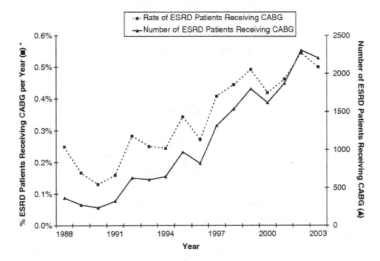

Figure 1. Graph depicting the increasing trend in the number of patients with end-stage renal disease (ESRD) under-going coronary artery bypass grafting (CABG) over a 15-year period (Data from Parikh DS, Swaminathan M, Archer LE, et al. Perioperative outcomes among patients with end-stage renal disease following coronary artery bypass surgery in the USA. Nephrol. Dial. Transpl 2010; 25(7):2275-2283).

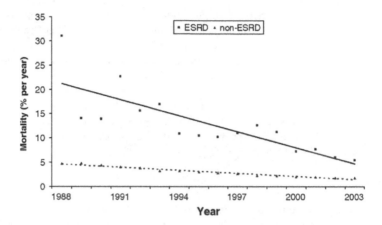

Figure 2. Graph depicting the constantly decreasing trend in mortality of patients with end-stage renal disease (ESRD) undergoing coronary artery bypass grafting (CABG) compared to patients without ESRD, over a 15-year period (Data from Parikh DS, Swaminathan M, Archer LE, et al. Perioperative outcomes among patients with end-stage renal disease following coronary artery bypass surgery in the USA. Nephrol. Dial. Transpl 2010; 25(7):2275-2283)..

Studies have shown that cardiovascular risk modification using ACC/AHA guideline recommended therapies for CAD, such as aspirin, beta blockers, hydroxymethyl coenzyme A (HMG-Co A inhibitors popularly known as statins) and angiotensin converting enzyme (ACE) inhibitors are used less frequently in patients with CKD when compared to patients without CKD [14,46-48]. These medications have been shown to decrease the risk of cardiovascular events across the population at risk. However, it is also true that many of those trials excluded patients with significant renal disease, which therefore poses a questions mark on their efficacy in patients with advanced CKD. Randomized trials to evaluate efficacy of these medications in patients with advanced renal dysfunction are warranted.

3. Peripheral arterial disease and CABG outcomes

The presence of peripheral arterial disease (PAD) plays a significant role in the potential morbidity and mortality of patients undergoing CABG. Coexisting CAD and PAD significantly influences long term survival adversely [49,50]. In the Coronary Artery Surgery Study (CASS), PAD was found to carry a higher risk of mortality even when compared to patients who had previously experienced myocardial infarction and angina [51].PAD is included as a major risk factor when calculating risk of mortality in patients undergoing CABG [1,2]. Non-invasive diagnostic testing for PAD includes segmental pressure measurement, treadmill stress, and Doppler ultrasound with the most significant information provided by the ankle-brachial index (ABI). Normally it is greater than 1.0 while <0.9 is considered abnormal. In patients with critical limb ischemia, the ABI is commonly <0.4. It is suspected that in PAD patients, poor surgical outcomes after CABG could be related to rapid progression of atherosclerotic coronary artery disease and more extensive small vessel

CAD with poor target foci for intervention resulting in higher mortality rates. Also the highly variable rates of CAD progression in patients with and without PAD leads to poor outcomes as well [52].

In comparison with PCI, CABG has been shown to improve mortality significantly more in patients with PAD. Data from 1305 consecutive patients undergoing coronary revascularization (PCI, n = 341; CABG, n = 964) between 1994 and 1996 showed that patients with PAD undergoing CABG had better survival at 3 years when compared to PCI (hazard ratio 0.68; 95% CI 0.46-1.00; p = 0.05) [53].

In a retrospective analysis on 1,164 consecutive patients who underwent CABG (370 with PAD), it was shown that PAD did not impact 30-day mortality. However, multivariable analysis showed that patients with PAD had a significantly worse 9-year survival rate compared to patients without PAD (72.9% vs. 82.8%; adjusted hazard ratio, 1.7; p = 0.004) [54]. Trachiotis et al studied long-term survival in 11,830 CABG patients, 744 of whom had LVEF <0.35. Among all patients, regardless of ventricular function, diabetes was linked with a 59% increase in the relative risk of death [55]. It was shown by Birkmeyer et al that patients undergoing CABG with history of PAD had a 20% five-year mortality rate as compared to 8% for those without known PAD [56,57]. Kaul et al showed that after risk factor adjustment, patients with PAD had mortality rates twice as high as patients without PAD [58]. Loponen et al showed in a multicenter study on 3000 patients that patients with PAD undergoing CABG had a 71% greater in-hospital mortality rate than those without PAD [59].

In a ten year prospective study of 8000 patients with PAD undergoing CABG, it was seen that they had a higher incidence of various intra- and post-operative complications including arrhythmias, stroke, pulmonary complications, low cardiac output state, longer hospital stay, infections, and acute renal failure. These results have been borne out by other studies as well [60-63].

The anatomic diversity of obstructive atherosclerotic disease process is particularly interesting. Patient can have isolated cerebrovascular disease involving carotid arteries, or lower extremity arterial disease or a combination thereof. It has been shown that as the number of involved arterial beds increases, the mortality increases. In a study on 2817 patients undergoing CABG, it was demonstrated that when compared to patients with CAD alone, the mortality was 1.6 times, 2.5 times, and 2.8 times higher for patients with concomitant cerebrovascular disease, lower extremity arterial disease and both cerebrovascular and lower extremity arterial disease, respectively [64]. Another study found that in patients younger than 40 years, the most common pattern of lower extremity arterial disease is aortoiliac disease while in patients older than 40 years, femoro-popliteal disease is predominant and causes intermittent claudication in 65% of these patients [65].

Commonly, patients with iliac disease have hemodynamically significant stenoses, while majority of patients with femoral disease have total occlusions characteristically involving long segments of the superficial femoral artery. Consequently, percutaneous revascularization of the femoral arterial segments is technically difficult as compared to iliac endovascular repair. The risk factors associated with PAD are similar to those for CAD, with diabetes and smoking being the major ones. Diabetes is a major predictor of outcomes of CABG in patients with PAD. It is associated with more than 50% of major amputations in patients with PAD. In a study of 261 patients by Jonason et al (47 diabetic and 224 non diabetic), at six year follow up, showed an incidence of gangrene in 31% of diabetics as compared to 5% in non-diabetics [66]. Also hypertension, strong family history of premature atherosclerotic vascular disease, and hyperlipidemia are also contributory. Progression to severe ischemia or amputation in symptomatic patients with intermittent claudication occurs at 1.4% per year with poor prognosis in patients with diabetes and smoking [66,67].

The rate of all-cause mortality in patients with large-vessel PAD compared with the normal population is three times greater, while the risk of cardiovascular mortality is six-fold more, with the most common etiology being myocardial infarction or stroke [67]. In an analysis of 900 patients with LVEF of 0.35 or less, among whom 38% were diabetics, all-cause mortality was 26% in diabetics and 24% in non-diabetics (p>0.05). However, 4 -year re-hospitalization rates were 85% in diabetics and 69% in non-diabetics (p = 0.0001). The incidence of superficial sternal wound infection was 3.3 times higher and of renal failure was 2.2 times greater in diabetic patients as compared to non- diabetics [68].

Finally, a combination of CKD and PAD is even worse for the overall outcomes of patients undergoing CABG. In a prospective study of 36,641 CABG patients over a ten year period, long term survival rates of patient groups stratified as non- diabetic, diabetic with PAD and CKD, and diabetics without PAD and CKD were determined. The follow up was equivalent to 154,140 person-years. Annual mortality rates for non-diabetic and diabetic groups were 3.1 deaths per 100 person-years and 4.4 deaths per 100 person-years, respectively. The annual mortality rate for diabetic subjects with CKD, PAD, or both was significantly higher at 9.4 deaths per 100 person-years. Thus, patients undergoing CABG who are diabetic along with having PAD and CKD are at highest mortality risk over long term follow up of 10 years [69].

3.1. Impact of cerebrovascular disease on outcomes of CABG

Carotid artery stenosis is an important risk factor in determining post CABG outcomes such as stroke and additionally, has a direct impact on perioperative mortality [70,71]. Duplex ultrasonography or contrast-based techniques can be utilized pre-operatively in high risk patients with age greater than 65 years and multiple risk factors such as diabetes mellitus, hypertension, and previous transient ischemic attacks or stroke. In case of severe carotid disease, surgical planning might need to include carotid endarterectomy along with CABG simultaneously versus consideration for endovascular repair of carotid disease pre-operatively.

In a study of 582 patients undergoing CABG, preoperative carotid artery duplex scans were performed to assess the presence of asymptomatic carotid artery stenosis. >50% uni- or bilateral stenosis was present in 22% while >80% uni- or bilateral stenosis was present in 12% of patients. The post-operative hemispheric stroke rate in patients with carotid stenosis >50% was 3.8% as compared to 0.34% in patients without carotid stenosis (p = 0.0072). Also the risk of hemispheric stroke was 5.3% in patients with unilateral 80% to 99% stenosis, or bilateral 50% to 99% stenosis, or unilateral occlusion with contralateral 50% or greater stenosis. Patients with a unilateral 50% to 79% stenosis did not suffer a stroke in this study [70].

In a study of 3344 patients undergoing CABG who were followed over a three year period to assess the effect of carotid artery stenosis on perioperative stroke and mortality, it was found that the clinical outcomes were directly related to the degree of carotid stenosis. Patients with carotid stenosis <60% had a significantly less risk of suffering perioperative stroke and mortality when compared to patients with >60% stenosis, especially patients with a totally occluded carotid artery [71].

These studies signify carotid artery disease as an important subset of patients with PAD which can adversely affect post CABG outcomes in terms of incidence of stroke and mortality rates.

3.2. Impact of microvascular disease on CABG

Microvascular disease, such as that which occurs in diabetic patients has also been shown to adversely affect outcomes after CABG. These complications generally stem from a cumulative poor glycemic control. In a study on 223 patients with diabetic retinopathy followed 11 years post-CABG, it was found that diabetic retinopathy was a strong independent predictor of overall mortality (relative risk [RR], 4.0), and repeat revascularization (RR, 3.0) [72].

3.3. Use of LIMA and SVG grafts

Use of internal mammary artery (IMA) grafts in patients undergoing CABG have been associated with improved short and long-term survival, increased patency and decreased perioperative mortality. However, in patients with significant PAD, it could be the major source of collateral flow to the lower extremities in patients with aorto-iliac disease. The finding that the mammary artery collateralized the iliac artery led to major treatment changes in all patients undergoing CABG [73]. Therefore, it is advisable to perform angiography of this conduit before referral for CABG in patients with PAD.

In a study on 21,873 patients among whom 87% underwent grafting of left IMA, and were followed for 7 years, there was a significantly decreased risk of mortality in all subgroups. Additionally, the incidence of stroke, repeat intervention, bleeding complications, mediastinitis or sternal dehiscence requiring surgery was less with use of IMA grafts. The adjusted mortality rate was 2.2% vs. 4.9%, and rate of stroke was 1.6% vs. 1.9% in patients undergoing IMA versus no IMA grafting, respectively. Infective mediastinitis or sternal dehiscence was seen in 1.1% of the LIMA group and 1.3% of the non-LIMA group [74].

It has been shown that use of LIMA grafts is even associated with lower in hospital mortality even in patients with a higher number of risk factors such as age greater than 70 years, elevated left ventricular end-diastolic pressure, left ventricular ejection fraction less than 40%, small body mass index, or clinical presentation in acute or emergency setting. So, there is a proven consistent trend of protective LIMA effect in high risk groups as well [75].

3.4. Impact of PAD on graft failure in CABG

A major cause of short-term mortality post CABG and therefore, poor surgical outcome is graft failure. In 1972, Lesperance et al reported that out of a total of 105 saphenous vein grafts (SVG) used during CABG, 20% had early occlusion [76]. In a review of SVG disease, Motwani and Topol showed an early SVG occlusion rate of 15% and elucidated the diverse etiology of SVG closure [77]. At one month post CABG, the major cause of graft failure is thrombosis. From a month to one year post CABG, intimal hyperplasia is the chief contributor while after one year, atherosclerotic changes have been primarily implicated. They also demonstrated that arterial runoff was the single most important determinant of short-term graft survival. Occluded vessels distal to the SVG anastomosis resulted in thrombosis and graft failures.

The internal diameter of the mid-LAD is approximately1.7 mm, while that of the saphenous vein is 4-5 mm. This difference leads to variable flow rates and slow flow velocity in the SVG as compared to mid-LAD. The sluggish flow causes red blood cell sledging and consequent thrombosis. The internal diameter of the IMA is almost equivalent the mid-LAD, and thus there is decreased risk of graft thrombosis. They also highlighted that LIMA graft in addition to matching favorable dimensions of native LAD, lacks valves, has less endothelial fenestrations, and has a greater resistance to trauma while it is being harvested [78]. Other advantageous physiological characteristics of the IMA include higher flow reserve and shear stress, greater nitric oxide and prostacyclin production leading to vasodilation and inhibition of platelet aggregation, appropriate relaxation response to thrombin, less vasoconstrictor sensitivity and high vasodilator sensitivity along with decreased number of fibroblast growth factor receptors thus reducing plaque formation [78].

In a patent population in whom both radial artery and SVG grafts were used for CABG, it was found that radial artery grafts fared worse than SVGs in patients with PAD [79].

3.5. Off pump CABG and standard CABG

Off pump CABG (OPCAB) is referred to as CABG without use of cardiopulmonary bypass or cardioplegia while on pump CABG is referred to the use of cardiopulmonary bypass and cardioplegia. There have been various studies which generally show benefits of OPCAB as compared to standard CABG. Benefits include less bleeding complications, stroke and renal failure after OPCAB.

In a retrospective analysis of 68,000 patients by Ractz et al, 9000 OPCAB revascularizations were performed with this group comprising many high-risk patients including those with >60 years of age, female gender, low LVEF, previous history of CABG, stroke, PAD, congestive heart failure, calcified aortic disease, and renal failure. It was seen that the standard CABG group as compared to OPCAB group had higher rates of stroke (2.0% vs. 1.6%), higher bleeding complications (2.2% vs. 1.6%), and prolonged hospital stay by one day. At 3-year follow-up, the need for repeat revascularization was also greater in standard CABG versus the OPCAB group [80].

In another retrospective study by Mack et al in which 17401 patients were reviewed and 7283 received OPCAB, it was found that even in patients with PAD among other risk factors, patients undergoing OPCAB had improved mortality when compared to patients undergoing on-pump CABG (1.9% vs. 3.5%). The rate of complications including major bleeding, wound infection, atrial fibrillation, permanent stroke, gastrointestinal and respiratory complications, renal failure, myocardial infarction, and multiorgan failure was higher in standard CABG group [81].

In another study comprising 214 patients at high risk (high EuroSCORE) with >50% of patients with significant PAD, it was found that off-pump CABG was safer and was associated with less early post-operative complications including multi-organ failure [82].

Patients with PAD are likely to have complex atheromatous plaques in the arch of aorta which poses a risk for peri-operative stroke during manipulation for on-pump CABG surgery An analysis of 422 patients demonstrated that there was a significant reduction in post-operative stroke in patients who had OPCAB when compared to patients undergoing on-pump surgery (0.9% vs. 5.7%, p=0.007) [83]. Therefore, for patients with PAD needing CABG, OPCAB would help avoid manipulation of aorta and in turn, decrease post-operative cerebrovascular complications.

Over a period of time, an increasing body of evidence has indicated that OPCAB is better than on-pump CABG, especially in high-risk groups. This includes a significant benefit of OPCAB in patients with PAD as it reduces the risk of postoperative stroke. As it has been shown in the SYNTAX trial, which is the largest contemporary trial comparing PCI versus CABG, showed that the major risk with CABG appears to be the increased risk of stroke from it [84]. OPCAB can, at least reduce that chance which might improve the overall benefit of CABG in patients with advanced CAD.

4. Conclusion

Based on current data, there is sufficient evidence to suggest that diabetes, peripheral arterial disease, CKD, on-pump CABG, increased aortic cross clamp and cardiopulmonary bypass duration, lack of use of IMA graft are strongly associated with poor in hospital, short term and long term outcomes after CABG. Rigorous modification of these risk factors to the maximum possible extent preoperatively can result in further improvement of surgical outcomes following CABG.

Author details

Muhammad A. Chaudhry[1], Zainab Omar[2] and Faisal Latif[3]

*Address all correspondence to: faisal-latif@ouhsc.edu

1 Scripps Green Hospital, La Jolla, California, USA

2 King Edward Medical College, Lahore, Pakistan

3 University of Oklahoma Health Sciences Center, Oklahoma City, Oklahoma, USA

References

[1] Roques F, Nashef SA, Michel P, Gauducheau E, de Vincentiis C, Baudet E, Cortina J, David M, Faichney A, Gabrielle F, Gams E, Harjula A, Jones MT, Pintor PP, Salamon R, Thulin L. Risk factors and outcome in European cardiac surgery: analysis of the EuroSCORE multinational database of 19030 patients. Eur J Cardiothorac Surg. 1999 Jun;15(6):816-22; discussion 822-3.

[2] Edwards FH, Grover FL, Shroyer AL, Schwartz M, Bero J, Clark RE. The Society of Thoracic Surgeons National Cardiac Surgery Database: current risk assessment Ann Thorac Surg 1997;63:903-908.

[3] Cockcroft DW, Gault MH. Prediction of creatinine clearance from serum creatinine. Nephron 1976;16 (1): 31–41.

[4] Levey AS, Bosch JP, Lewis JB, Greene T, Rogers N, Roth D. A more accurate method to estimate glomerular filtration rate from serum creatinine: a new prediction equation. Modification of Diet in Renal Disease Study Group. Annals of Internal Medicine 1999;130 (6): 461–70.

[5] Manjunath G, Tighiouart H, Ibrahim H, MacLeod B, Salem DN, Griffith JL, Coresh J, Levey AS, Sarnak MJ. Level of kidney function as a risk factor for atherosclerotic cardiovascular outcomes in the community. J Am Coll Cardiol. 2003; 41(1):47-55.

[6] Strippoli GF, Craig JC, Manno C, et al. Hemoglobin targets for the anemia of chronic kidney disease: a meta-analysis of randomized, controlled trials. J Am Soc Nephrol 2004; 15: 3154-3165.

[7] Cozzolino M, Brancaccio D, Gallieni M, et al. Pathogenesis of vascular calcification in chronic kidney disease. Kidney Int 2005;68: 429-436.

[8] Levin A, Li YC. Vitamin D and its analogues: do they protect against cardiovascular disease in patients with kidney disease? Kidney Int. 2005 Nov; 68(5):1973-81.

Impact of Renal Dysfunction and Peripheral Arterial Disease on Post-Operative Outcomes After
Coronary Artery Bypass Grafting

127

[9] Agirbasli M, Weintraub WS, Chang GL, et al.Outcome of coronary revascularization in patients on renal dialysis. Am J Cardiol 2000;86:395-399.

[10] Labrousse L, de Vincentiis C, Madonna F, et al. Early and long term results of coronary artery bypass grafts in patients with dialysis dependent renal failure. Eur J Cardiothorac Surg 1999;15:691-696.

[11] Ivens K, Gradaus F, Heering P, et al. Myocardial revascularization in patients with end-stage renal disease: comparison of percutaneous transluminal coronary angioplasty and coronary artery bypass grafting. Int Urol Nephrol 2001; 32: 717-723.

[12] Kahn JK, Rutherford BD, McConahay DR, et al.Short- and long-term outcome of percutaneous transluminal coronary angioplasty in chronic dialysis patients. Am Heart J 1990;119:484-489.

[13] Schoebel F, Gradaus F, Ivens K, Heering P, Jax TW, Grabensee B, Strauer B, Leschke M. Restenosis after elective coronary balloon angioplasty in patients with end stage renal disease: a case-control study using quantitative coronary angiography. Heart. 1997; 78(4): 337-342.

[14] Latif F, Kleiman NS, Cohen DJ, Pencina MJ, Yen CH, Cutlip DE, Moliterno DJ, Nassif D, Lopez JJ, Saucedo JF; EVENT Investigators. In-hospital and 1-year outcomes among percutaneous coronary intervention patients with chronic kidney disease in the era of drug-eluting stents: a report from the EVENT (Evaluation of Drug Eluting Stents and Ischemic Events) registry. JACC Cardiovasc Interv. 2009;2(1):37-45.

[15] Herzog CA, Ma JZ, Collins AJ. A comparative survival of dialysis patients in the United States after coronary angioplasty, coronary artery stenting, and coronary artery bypass grafting and impact of diabetes. Circulation 2002;106:2207-11.

[16] Hillis GS, Croal BL, Buchan KG, et al. Renal function and outcome from coronary artery bypass grafting: Impact on mortality after a 2.3-year follow up. Circulation 2006; 113:1056-1062.

[17] Cooper WA, O'Brien SM, Thourani VH, et al. Impact of renal dysfunction on outcomes of coronary artery bypass surgery: Results from the Society of Thoracic Surgeons National Adult Cardiac Database. Circulation 2006; 113:1063-1070.

[18] Liu JY, Birkmeyer NJ, Sanders JH, et al. Risks of morbidity and mortality in dialysis patients undergoing coronary artery bypass surgery. Circulation. 2000; 102: 2973-2977.

[19] Zoccali C, Ciccarili M, Maggiori Q. Defective reflex control of heart rate in dialysis patients: evidence for an autonomic afferent lesion. Clin Sci Mol Med 1982;63: 285-292.

[20] Charytan DM, Yang SS, McGurk S, Rawn J. Long and short-term outcomes following coronary artery bypass grafting in patients with and without chronic kidney disease. Nephrol. Dial. Transplant 2010; 25(11): 3654-3663.

[21] Zhong H, David T, Zhang AH, Fang W, Ahmad M, Bargman JM, Oreopoulos DG. Coronary artery bypass grafting in patients on maintenance dialysis: is peritoneal dialysis a risk factor of operative mortality? Int Urol Nephrol. 2009; 41(3):653-62.

[22] Hamada Y, Kawachi K, Nakata T, Takano S, Tsunooka N, Sato M, Watanabe Y, Nakano N, Miyauchi K, Kohtani T. Cardiac surgery in patients with end-stage renal disease. Utility of continuous ambulatory peritoneal dialysis. Jpn J Thorac Cardiovasc Surg. 2001 Feb; 49(2):99-102.

[23] Herlitz J, Wognsen GB, Karlson BW, et al. Mortality, mode of death and risk indicators for death during 5 years after coronary artery bypass grafting among patients with and without a history of diabetes mellitus. Coron Artery Dis. 2000; 11:339–346.

[24] Clough RA, Leavitt BJ, Morton JR, et al. The effect of comorbid illness on mortality outcomes in cardiac surgery. Arch Surg. 2002; 137: 428–432.

[25] Szabo Z, Hakanson E, Svedjeholm R. Early postoperative outcome and medium-term survival in 540 diabetic and 2239 non-diabetic patients undergoing coronary artery bypass grafting. Ann Thorac Surg. 2002; 74: 712–719.

[26] Thourani VH, Weintraub WS, Stein B, et al. Influence of diabetes mellitus on early and late outcome after coronary artery bypass grafting. Ann Thorac Surg. 1999; 67: 1045–1052.

[27] Morris JJ, Smith LR, Jones RH, et al. Influence of Diabetes and Mammary Artery Grafting on Survival after Coronary Bypass. Circulation. 1991; Suppl III: III-275–III-284.

[28] Stevens LM, Carrier M, Perrault LP, Hébert Y, Cartier R, Bouchard D, Fortierand A, Pellerin M. Influence of diabetes and bilateral internal thoracic artery grafts on long-term outcome for multivessel coronary artery bypass grafting.. Eur J Cardiothorac Surg (2005) 27 (2): 281-288.

[29] Salomon NW, Page US, Okies JE, Stephens J, Krause AH, Bigelow JC.Diabetes mellitus and coronary artery bypass. Short-term risk and long-term prognosis. J Thorac Cardiovasc Surg 1983; 85(2):264-271.

[30] Jacoby RM, Nesto RW. Acute myocardial infarction in the diabetic patient: pathophysiology, clinical course and prognosis. J Am Coll Cardiol 1992;20(3):736-744.

[31] OsendeJI, Badimon JJ, Fuster V, Herson P, Rabito P, Vidhun R, Zaman A, Rodriguez OJ, Lev EI, Rauch U, Heflt G, Fallon JT, Crandall JP. Blood thrombogenicity in type 2 diabetes mellitus patients is associated with glycemic control. J Am Coll Cardiol 2001;38(5):1307-1312.

[32] Williams SB, Cusco JA, Roddy MA, Johnstone MT, Creager MA. Impaired nitric oxide-mediated vasodilation in patients with non-insulin-dependent diabetes mellitus. J Am Coll Cardiol 1996; 27(3):567-574.

[33] Isolated Systolic Hypertension Is Associated with Adverse Outcomes from Coronary Artery Bypass Grafting Surgery. Solomon Aronson, Denis Boisvert, William Lapp.A & A May 2002 vol. 94 no. 5 1079-1084.

[34] Cheung AK, Sarnak MJ, Yan G, Dwyer JT, Heyka RJ, Rocco MV, Teehan BP, Levey AS. Atherosclerotic cardiovascular disease risks in chronic hemodialysis patients. Kidney Int. 2000 Jul;58(1):353-62.

[35] Shoji T, Nishizawa Y, Kawagishi T, Tanaka M, Kawasaki K, Tabata T, Inoue T, Morii H. Atherogenic lipoprotein changes in the absence of hyperlipidemia in patients with chronic renal failure treated by hemodialysis. Atherosclerosis. 1997 Jun; 131(2): 229-36.

[36] Ross R. Atherosclerosis-An inflammatory disease. N Engl J Med1999;340:115-26.

[37] Schettler V, Wieland E, Methe H, Schuff-Werner P, Müller GA. Oxidative stress during dialysis: effect on free radical scavenging enzyme (FRSE) activities and glutathione (GSH) concentration in granulocytes. Nephrol. Dial. Transpl 1998; 13(10): 2588-2593.

[38] Conlon PJ, Crowley J, Stack R, Neary JJ, Stafford-Smith M, White WD, Newman MF, Landolfo K. Renal artery stenosis is not associated with the development of acute renal failure following coronary artery bypass grafting. Ren Fail. 2005; 27(1):81-6.

[39] Erentug V, Bozbuga N, Polat A, Tuncer A, Sareyyupoglu B, Kirali K, Akinci E, Yakut C. Coronary bypass procedures in patients with renal artery stenosis. J Card Surg. 2005; 20(4):345-9.

[40] Anderson RJ, O'brien M, MaWhinney S, VillaNueva CB, Moritz TE, Sethi GK, Henderson WG, Hammermeister KE, Grover FL, Shroyer AL. Renal failure predisposes patients to adverse outcome after coronary artery bypass surgery. VA Cooperative Study #5. Kidney Int. 1999 Mar; 55(3):1057-62.

[41] Winkelmayer WC, Levin R, Avorn J. Chronic kidney disease as a risk factor for bleeding complications after coronary artery bypass surgery. Am J Kidney Dis 2003;41: 84-89.

[42] Jennings RB, Reimer KA. The cell biology of acute myocardial ischemia. Annu Rev Med, 1991; 42:225-46.

[43] Doenst T, Borger MA, Weisel RD, Yau TM, Maganti M, Rao V. Relation between aortic cross-clamp time and mortality — not as straightforward as expected. Eur J Cardiothorac Surg 2008; 33(4):660-665.

[44] Rastan AJ, Eckenstein JI, Hentschel B, Funkat AK, Gummert JF, Doll N, Walther T, Falk V, Mohr FW. Emergency Coronary Artery Bypass Graft Surgery for Acute Coronary Syndrome Beating Heart Versus Conventional Cardioplegic Cardiac Arrest Strategies. Circulation. 2006; 114: I-477-485.

[45] Parikh DS, Swaminathan M, Archer LE, Inrig JK, Szczech LA, Shaw AD, Patel UD. Perioperative outcomes among patients with end-stage renal disease following coronary artery bypass surgery in the USA. Nephrol. Dial. Transpl 2010; 25(7):2275-2283.

[46] Wright RS, Reeder GS, Herzog CA, et al. Acute myocardial infarction and renal dysfunction: a high-risk combination. Ann Intern Med. 2002; 137:563–570.

[47] Best PJ, Lennon R, Ting HH, Bell MR, Rihal CS, Holmes DR, Berger PB. The impact of renal insufficiency on clinical outcomes in patients undergoing percutaneous coronary interventions. J Am Coll Cardiol 2002;39(7):1113-9.

[48] Smith SC, Benjamin EJ, Bonow RO, et al. AHA/ACCF Secondary Prevention and Risk Reduction Therapy for Patients With Coronary and Other Atherosclerotic Vascular Disease: 2011 Update: Title and subTitle Break A Guideline From the American Heart Association and American College of Cardiology Foundation Endorsed by the World Heart Federation and the Preventive Cardiovascular Nurses Association. J Am Coll Cardiol. 2011;58(23):2432-2446.

[49] Casser A, Poldermans D, Rihal CS, Gersch BJ. The management of combined coronary artery disease and peripheral vascular disease. European Heart Journal 2010;31(13):1565–1572.

[50] Steg G, Bhatt DL, Wilson PWF, D'Agostino R, Ohman M, Rother J, et al. for the REACH registry investigators one-year cardiovascular event rates in outpatients with atherothrombosis. The Journal of the American Medical Association, 297 (11) (2007), pp. 1197–1206

[51] Eagle KA, Rihal CS, Foster ED, Mickel MC, Gersch BJ for the Coronary Artery Surgery Study (CASS) investigators. Long-term survival in patients with coronary artery disease: importance of peripheral vascular disease. J Am Coll Cardiol 1994;23(5): 1091–1095.

[52] Shub C, Vlietstra RE, Smith HC, Fulton RE, Elveback LR. The unpredictable progression of symptomatic coronary artery disease: a serial clinical-angiographic analysis Mayo Clin Proc 1981; 56:155-160.

[53] O'Rourke DJ, Quinton HB, Piper W, Hernandez F, Morton J, Hettleman B, et al. Survival in patients with peripheral vascular disease after percutaneous coronary intervention and coronary artery bypass graft surgery. The Annals of Thoracic Surgery 2004;78(2): 466–470.

[54] Chu D, Bakaeen FG, Wang XL, Dao TK, LeMaire SA, Coselli JS, Huh J. The Impact of peripheral vascular disease on long-term survival after Coronary Artery Bypass Graft Surgery. Ann Thorac Surg. 2008;86(4):1175-80.

[55] Trachiotis GD, Weintraub WS, Johnston TS, Jones EL, Guyton RA, Craver JM. Coronary artery bypass grafting in patients with advanced left ventricular dysfunction, Ann Thorac Surg 1998;66:1632-1639.

[56] Birkmeyer JD, O'Connor GT, Quinton HB. et al. The effect of peripheral vascular disease on in-hospital mortality rates with coronary artery bypass surgery. J Vasc Surg
1995; 21445- 452.

[57] Birkmeyer JD, Quinton HB, O'Connor NJ. et al. The effect of peripheral vascular disease on long-term mortality after coronary artery bypass surgery. Arch Surg
1996;131316- 321.

[58] Kaul TK, Fields BL, Wyatt DA, Jones CR, Kahn DR. Surgical management in patients
with coexistent coronary and cerebrovascular disease: long-term results. Chest 1994;
1061349-1357.

[59] Loponen P, Taskinen P, Laakkonen E. et al. Peripheral vascular disease as predictor
of outcome after coronary artery bypass grafting. Scand J Surg 2002;91160- 165.

[60] Criqui MH, Langer RD, Fronek A, et al. Mortality over a period of 10 years in patients with peripheral arterial disease. N Engl J Med. 1992; 326: 381–386.

[61] Minakata K, Konishi Y, Matsumoto M, Aota M, Sugimoto A, Nonaka M, et al. Influence of peripheral vascular occlusive disease on the morbidity and mortality of coronary artery bypass grafting. Japanese Circulation Journal 2000;64(12):905–908.

[62] Collison T, Smith JM, Engel AM. Peripheral vascular disease and outcomes following
coronary artery bypass graft surgery. Archives of Surgery 2006;141(12):1214–1218.

[63] Cooper EA, Edelman B, Wilson MK, Bannon PG, Vallely MP. Off-pump Coronary
Artery Bypass Grafting in Elderly and High-risk Patients – A Review. Heart Lung
and Circulation 2011;20(11):694-703.

[64] Pokorski RJ. Effect Of Peripheral Vascular Disease On Long-Term Mortality After
Coronary Artery Bypass Graft Surgery. Journal of Insurance Medicine 1997,
29:192-194.

[65] Krajewski LP, Olin JW. Atherosclerosis of the aorta and lower-extremity arteries. In:
Young JR, Olin JW, Bartholomew JR, eds. Peripheral Vascular Diseases. St Louis, Mo:
Mosby-Year Book, Inc; 1996:208–233.

[66] Jonason T, Bergstrom R. Cessation of smoking in patients with intermittent claudication: effects on the risk of peripheral vascular complications, myocardial infarction
and mortality. Acta Med Scand. 1987;221: 253–260.

[67] DeBakey ME, Glaeser DH. Patterns of atherosclerosis: effect of risk factors on recurrence and survival-analysis of 11,890 cases with more than 25-year follow-up. Am J
Cardiol. 2000;85: 1045–1053.

[68] Whang W, Bigger JT. Diabetes and outcomes of coronary artery bypass graft surgery
in patients with severe left ventricular dysfunction: results from The CABG Patch
Trial database. J Am Coll Cardiol. 2000; 36(4):1166-1172.

[69] Leavitt BJ, Sheppard L, Maloney C, et al. Effect of Diabetes and Associated Condi-
      tions on Long-Term Survival After Coronary Artery Bypass Graft Surgery. Circula-
      tion. 2004;110(11 Suppl 1):I-I41-4.

[70] Schwartz LB, Bridgman AH, Kieffer RW, Wilcox RA, McCann RL, Tawil MP, Scott
      SM. Asymptomatic carotid artery stenosis and stroke in patients undergoing cardio-
      pulmonary bypass. J Vasc Surg. 1995; 21(1):146-53.

[71] Tunio AM, Hingorani A, Ascher E. The impact of an occluded internal carotid artery
      on the mortality and morbidity of patients undergoing coronary artery bypass graft-
      ing. Am J Surg. 1999; 178(3):201-5

[72] Ono T, Kobayashi J, Sasako Y, Bando K, Tagusari O, Niwaya K, Imanaka H, Nakata-
      ni T, Kitamura S. The impact of diabetic retinopathy on long-term outcome following
      coronary artery bypass graft surgery. J Am Coll Cardiol. 2002;40(3):428-36.

[73] Ben-Dor I, Waksman R, Satler LF, Bernardo N, Torguson R, Li Y, Gonzalez MA, Ma-
      luenda G, Weissman G, Hanna NN, Monath A, Gallino R, Lindsay J, Kent KM, Pi-
      chard AD. A further word of caution before using the internal mammary artery for
      coronary revascularization in patients with severe peripheral vascular disease! Cath-
      eter Cardiovasc Interv. 2010 Feb 1;75(2):195-201.

[74] Leavitt BJ, O'Connor GT, Olmstead EM, Morton JR, Maloney CT, Dacey LJ, Hernan-
      dez F, Lahey SJ. Use of the Internal Mammary Artery Graft and In-Hospital Mortali-
      ty and Other Adverse Outcomes Associated With Coronary Artery Bypass Surgery;
      Circulation. 2001; 103: 507-512.

[75] Cosgrove DM, Loop FD, Lytle BW, et al. Does mammary artery grafting increase sur-
      gical risk? Circulation. 1985;72:II-170–II-174.

[76] Lesperance J, Bourassa MG, Biron P, et al. Aorta to coronary artery saphenous vein
      grafts: preoperative angiographic criteria for successful surgery. Am J Cardiol.
      1972;30: 459–465.

[77] Motwani JG, Topol EJ. Aortocoronary saphenous vein graft disease: pathogenesis,
      predisposition, and prevention. Circulation. 1998; 97:916–931.

[78] O'Connor NJ, Morton JR, Birkmeyer JD, et al. Effect of coronary artery diameter in
      patients undergoing coronary bypass surgery: the Northern New England Cardio-
      vascular Disease Study Group. Circulation. 1996; 93: 652–655.

[79] Hata M, Yoshitake I, Wakui S, Unosawa S, Kimura H, Hata H, Shiono M. Long-term
      patency rate for radial artery vs. saphenous vein grafts using same-patient materials.
      Circ J. 2011;75(6):1373-7.

[80] Racz MJ, Hannan EL, Isom OW, Subramanian VA, Jones RH, Gold JP, Ryan TJ, Hart-
      man A, Culliford AT, Bennett E, Lancey RA, Rose EA. A comparison of short- and
      long-term outcomes after off-pump and on-pump coronary artery bypass graft sur-
      gery with sternotomy. J Am Coll Cardiol. 2004; 43: 557–564.

[81] Mack MJ, Pfister A, Bachand D, Emery R, Magee MJ, Connolly M, Subramanian VA. Comparison of coronary bypass surgery with and without cardiopulmonary bypass in patients with multivessel disease. J Thorac Cardiovasc Surg. 2004; 127: 167–173.

[82] Munos E, Calderon J, Pillois X, Lafitte S, Ouattara A, Labrousse L, Roques X, Barandon L. Beating-heart coronary artery bypass surgery with the help of mini extracorporeal circulation for very high-risk patients. Perfusion. 2011;26(2):123-31.

[83] Karthik S, Musleh G, Grayson AD, Keenan DJM, Pullan DM, Dihmis WC, et al. Coronary surgery in patients with peripheral vascular disease: effect of avoiding cardiopulmonary bypass. The Annals of Thoracic Surgery, 77 (4) (2004), pp. 1245–1249.

[84] Serruys PW, Morice MC, Kappetein AP, et al. for the SYNTAX Investigators. Percutaneous Coronary Intervention versus Coronary-Artery Bypass Grafting for Severe Coronary Artery Disease. N Engl J Med 2009; 360:961-972.

Chapter 8

The Role of The Angiosome Model in Treatment of Critical Limb Ischemia

Kim Houlind and Johnny Christensen

Additional information is available at the end of the chapter

1. Introduction

Critical limb ischemia (CLI) is the major cause of amputation in the developed world but revascularization offers an opportunity for limb salvage. Revascularization can be performed either by bypass surgery or by endovascular techniques. Peripheral bypass surgery can be performed using artificial grafts, but vein grafts offer better limb salvage and graft patency [1].

When performing revascularization of the lower limb, common clinical practice and recent guidelines include grafting of the" best vessel" which crosses the level of the ankle in order to restore pulsatile flow to the foot [1]. This may lead to either direct perfusion of the ischemic area or – very often – indirect perfusion relying on collaterals surrounding the diseased zone. This strategy is different from the one used e.g. in coronary artery bypass surgery, where the aim is "complete revascularization" i.e. performing bypasses to every diseased vascular territory [2].

The arterial connections between different parts of the foot may quite often not be sufficient to ensure healing and to prevent amputation. For instance, approximately 15% of heel ulcers do not heal despite an open bypass graft to the dorsal pedal artery [3]

An alternative strategy, called the angiosome model, is based on the pioneering work of Taylor and coworkers [4], who, in the eighties, performed detailed dissections with injection of dye in the vessels. They demonstrated the fact that the body consists of "angiosomes" i.e. three-dimensional blocks of tissue perfused and drained by specific arterial and venous bundles. In a later report from the same group, the angiosomes of the leg and foot were described in detail [5]

Perfusion and drainage can occur between angiosomes by means of connecting "choke" vessels, but this perfusion is less effective than direct supply from the specific feed artery of the angiosome. It is worth noting that the choke vessels are diseased in patients with diabetes and atherosclerosis. This angiosome has had profound impact on the developement of strategies for plastic and reconstructive surgery. However, only little attention has been paid to the angiosome model in treatment of critical limb ischemia. According to the angiosome model, the specific feed artery – rather than the "best vessel" – should be favoured for revascularization. The foot and ankle area consist of six angiosomes.

During the last few years, some studies have compared the results of "best vessel" versus "angiosome" directed revascularization. The studies include comparisons of both arterial bypass and percutaneous revascularization based on the two principles

This chapter aims at describing the role of the angiosome model in critical limb ischemia, and to review the current literature.

2. Anatomy

Blood supply to the foot is derived from the three tibial vessels, the Anterior tibial artery, the Posterior tibial artery, and the Peroneal artery. These three arteries give rise to six end-arteries, each supplying an angiosome (Figure 1).

1. The anterior tibial artery supplies the anterior ankle and continues as the dorsalis pedis artery, which supplies the dorsum of the foot. It gives off the lateral tarsal artery and branches into the first dorsal interosseal artery and the arcuate artery supplying the 2-4 interosseal arteries. It has been pointed out that the dorsalis pedis artery is extremely attenuated or absent in 12% of cases [6].

   The posterior tibial artery divides into three main branches:

2. The calcaneal branch, which arborizes into multiple braches, that supply the medial and plantar portion of the heel,

3. the medial plantar artery, supplying the medial, plantar part of the foot. Its boundaries encompass the instep, and, depending on anatomic variability, can include the hallux.

4. the lateral plantar artery which supplies the lateral midfoot as well as the entire plantar forefoot through the 4 plantar metatarsal arteries that emanate from the deep plantar arch. Normally, this angiosome also includes the plantar aspect of the hallux, depending on anatomic variability.

   The peroneal artery bifurcates into

5. the anterior perforating brach, supplying the lateral anterior upper ankle and

6. a calcaneal branch, supplying the lateral and plantar heel. Together with the calcaneal brach of the posterior tibila artery this artery ensures a double blood supply to the plantar aspect of the heel.

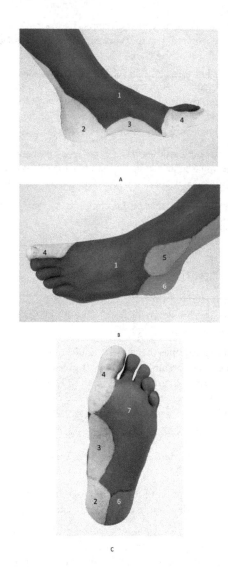

1. Dorsalis pedis angiosome
2. Medial calcaneal artery angiosome
3. Medial plantar artery angiosome
4. The hallux, which may be supplied by the feeding arteries of angiosomes 1, 2, or 6
5. Anterior perforating branch angiosome
6. Lateral calcaneal branch angiosome
7. Lateral plantar artery angiosome

Figure 1. Angiosomes shown on the surface of the foot. A. Medial view, B. Dorso-lateral view, C. Plantar view.

3. Interconnections

A number of interconnections exist between the angiosomes. When present, these interconnections exist *a priori* and – in contrast to the choke vessels described below - do not need a period of ischemia to open. However, as peripheral arterial disease progresses, these connections may be blocked.

The arterial-arterial connections include:

Anterior tibial to peroneal:

The lateral malleolar artery joins with the anterior perforating branch of the peroneal artery just above the ankle joint (Figure 2A).

Anterior tibial to posterior tibial:

The lateral plantar artery forms the deep plantar arch crossing the proximal 2,3, and 4th metatarsals and finally anastomoses directly with the dorsalis pedis artery in the first interspace (Figures 2A and 2B). The superficial and deep medial plantar arteries join at the cruciate anastomosis. Depending on what arteries predominate at or around the cruciate anastomosis, the hallux may be primarily nourished by the lateral plantar artery, medial plantar artery, the first dorsal metatarsal artery or simultaneously by either two or three of these arteries [7].

The medial plantar artery also interconnects with the anterior tibial tree as cutaneous branches connect proximally with medial branches of the dorsalis pedis artery and distally with branches of the first dorsal metatarsal artery.

Peroneal and posterior tibial connections:

Between one and three communicating branches between the peroneal artery and the posterior tibial artery proximal to the ankle joint deep to the Achilles tendon.

On the other hand, no direct arterial-arterial connection exists between the medial and lateral calcaneal arteries, which both supply the plantar aspect of the heel.

4. Choke vessels

Where no "true" arterial-arterial connections are present between neighbouring angiosomes, a network of reduced caliber "choke vessels" form a link. These vessels are normally inadequate to perfuse the area of a distant angiosome but may be provoked to dilate.

This is the theoretical base of the "delay phenomenon" which has been applied in plastic surgery. While the choke vessels between angiosomes in a skin or muscle flap may be sufficient to perfuse an adjacent vascular territory, necrosis will ususally appear in the choke vessel zone defining the next vascular territory. When designing a skin or muscle flap larger than two angiosomes, a two stage procedure might be performed. In the first stage, the perforators of the neighbouring angiosomes are ligated, causing the choke vessels between neighbouring angiosomes to dilate over a period of 4-10 days. After this delay period, a larger flap can be safely elevated [8]. There is good clinical and experimental evidence that this principle works for the transfer of skin grafts from essentially normal donor sites. These results may, however, not be extrapolated to other situations e.g. in the ischemic foot where distal, aggressive macroangiopathy is associated with microcirculatory changes like thrombosis, neuropathy, local sepsis, arterio-venous shunting and hypercoagulability [9].

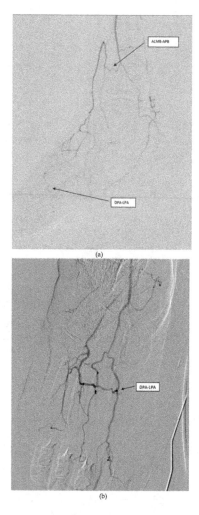

(a)

(b)

Figure 2. A. Lateral oblique projection of the anterior pedal vessels of a patient with peripheral occlusive arterial disease and patent arterial-arterial connections. ALMB-APB: Connection between the anterior lateral malleolar branch of the anterior tibial artery and the anterior perforating branch of the peroneal artery. DPA-LPA: Perforating branch connecting the dorsal pedal artery with the lateral plantar artery. B. Antero-posterior projection of the perforating branch connecting the dorsal pedal artery with the lateral plantar artery (DPA-LPA).

5. Imaging and assessment

5.1. Angiography

A fundamental prerequisite of providing angiosome-directed revascularization is profound knowledge of the anatomy of the pedal vasculature as well as adequate imaging technique including intraprocedural angiography of both tibial and pedal arteries. Manzi and coworkers have recently reported their experience from more than 2500 antegrade interventional procedures in patients with critical limb ischemia and diabetes [10]. For imaging of the pedal arteries they stress that prolonged filming is often necessary to record delayed enhancement of of pedal vessels from retrograde or collateral circulation and that both standard anteroposterior and lateral oblique projections should be obtained. They have established the following two criteria for correct positioning of the image intensifier: 1) The base of the fifth metatarsal bone must be seen to project outward from the base of the foot in the lateral oblique view and 2) the first proximal metatarsal interspace must be clearly visualized in the anteroposterior view. These two views tend to give a good overview of the pedal arteries and collaterals.

5.2. Doppler ultrasound

Attinger and coworkers have described in detail how to map the arterial-arterial connections using a Doppler device [7].

As an example, the Doppler signal is located from the posterior tibial artery over the tarsal tunnel. If the signal persists when occluding (by digital compression) the artery distally, there is antegrade flow along the posterior tibila artery. If the signal disappears, the flow is retrograde from the anterior tibial artery via the dorsalis pedis and lateral plantar arteries. Similarly, Doppler signal can be obtained from the anterior perforating branch of the peroneal artery in the lateral soft area between the tibia and fibula just above the ankle joint. When the anterior tibial artery is occluded at the takeoff of the lateral malleolar branch, the Doppler signal will persist if there is antegrade flow along the anterior perforating branch of the peroneal artery. If the Doppler signal disappears, filling of the anterior perforating branch must be retrograde from the anterior tibial artery through the lateral malleolar branch. The authors describe how the competence of these connections can have profound significance for the healing potential of an amputation wound.

5.3. Thermography

Nagase and coworkers [11] reported the results of plantar thermography of skin temperature in 129 non-ulcer diabetic patients and 32 normal volunteers. From the pattern of four different plantar angiosomes originally described by Attinger [7], they defined twenty different patterns of temperature distribution. The most common pattern in normal subjects was a "bilateral butterfly pattern" in which the medial arch showed the highest temperature (46.9%) or an even distribution of temperature across the entire planta of the feet (20.3%).

Recordings of the diabetic feet showed a lower proportion of feet with a "bilateral butterfly pattern" (13.9%), higher proportions of even distribution of temperature (39.1%) and a generally more diverse distribution of patterns in the rest. Although interesting, the study did not provide comparisons with angiographic findings that could confirm a correlation between the distribution of skin temperature and the distribution of lesions of feed arteries to the relevant angiosomes.

6. Results from direct versus indirect revascularization

A number of studies have been performed comparing the results of direct revascularization to the relevant angiosome with those of indirect revascularization either through collaterals or choke vessels.

In 2009, Neville and coworkers published a retrospective analysis of 43 patients undergoing bypass surgery for tissue loss due to ischemia [12]. Twenty-two were directly revascularized to the relevant agniosome while 21 were indirectly revascularized. Healing occurred in 91% of the directly revascularized patients and only 62% of the indirectly revascularized patients (p=0.03]. Major patient characteristics such as diabetes, tobacco use, and renal failure were evenly distributed between the directly revascularized and indirectly revascularized groups, but wound characteristics and infection were not reported.

On the other hand, Azuma and coworkers [13] reviewed the results of 249 consecutive distal bypasses for critical limb ischemia. 218 limbs were included in the initial analysis which proved significantly lower wound healing rate in the indirect revascularization group than in the direct revascularization group. This was especially the case in a subgroup of patients with end stage renal failure. This finding was, however, compromised by significant baseline differences between the groups especially characterized by a higher proportion of patients with heel ulcers and gangraene in the indirect revascularization group. After applying propensity scored analysis including only 48 pairs of limbs, the healing rate between the two groups did not reach statistical significance (p=0.185). The authors concluded that the angiosome concept was not relevant for open surgical treatment of critical limb ischemia in patients without end stage renal failure. This conclusion may be questioned in view of the limited statistical strength of the propensity scored analysis.

Iida and coworkers reviewed the results of endovascular treatment of 203 limbs in 177 consecutive patients with critical limb ischemia, Rutherford 5 or 6 [14]. During up to 4 years follow up, they found significantly higher limb salvage rate in patients with the directly revascularized than indirectly revascularized wounds. Interestingly, the total number of tibial vessels with run off did not influence the limb salvage rate in neither group, indicating that it is not important how much blood can be provided to the foot but rather whether i t reaches the ischemic area. In a later review by the same group [15], including 369 limbs from 329 consecutive patients, including only patients with isolated below-the-knee lesions, patients who had received direct revascularization experienced significantly higher levels of amputation-free survival and freedom from major adverse limb events than patients in whom only indirect revascularization was possible. In this review the finding was confirmed after propensity matching of groups. In multivariate analysis, elevated levels of c-reactive protein were found to be independent predictors of major amputation in the indirect revascularization group but not in the direct revascularization group. This may imply that indirect revascularization may be inadequate for the healing of infected wounds.

Alexandriescu and collegues have published several reports describing their experience with targeted primary angioplasty of diabetic foot lesions [16-17]. In a series of 124 limbs (98 patients), they were able to achieve direct revascularization in 82% [16]. Limb salvage was 91% at 12 months and 84% at three years follow-up. More recently, they published a historical comparison between their results before and after 2005 when they introduced the angiosome concept in their practice. Despite similar graft patency and technical success, they experienced a significantly better wound healing rate and limb preservation in the group of patients treated according to the angiosome concept [18]. This result is interesting although it is probably biased by the general learning curve of the group.

In a paper published together with Alexandriescu, the vascular surgery department at the University Hospital in Helsinki, Finland recently reported their results from the last three years [19]. In a population including approximately the same number of direct and indirect endovascular revascularizations, they found 74% of the wounds to have healed within one year in the directly revascularized group compared to 46% in the indirectly revascularizd group (p=0.002). The number of patients was, however, not reported.

Two studies, one surgical by Deguchi [20] and one endovascular by Blanes Ortí [21] failed to show any difference in wound healing time or limb salvage between directly or indirectly revascularized patients. Due to small numbers, the statistical strengh of these comparisons is, however, limited.

6.1. The influence of collaterals

The prognostic significance of indirect revascularization via collaterals was studied by Varela in a mixed cohort of venous bypass and endovascular treated patients with ischemic wounds [22]. Defining collaterals visible on perioperative angiograms, either between distal calcaneal peroneal branches and anterior or posterior tibial artery (n=16) or patent pedal arch connecting dorsal and plantar blood supply (n=2), they found a similar wound healing rate for indirect revascularization of the wound area through collaterals as for direct revascularization to the angiosome specific feed artery (92% versus 88% wound healing at 12 months follow-up). When including indirect revascularizations without visible collaterals, only 73% of the wounds had healed after 12 months (p=0.008).

6.2. The significance of venosomes

Anatomically, the venous drainage follows the arterial perfusion of the angiosomes [23] and Alexandriescu used the term venosome, when reporting the results of surgical deep calf vein arterialization. In a series of 26 limbs in 25 diabetic patients with very advanced below the knee occlusive disease, a PTFE bypass was made between an arterial inflow and a deep calf vein followed by selective embolization of collaterals, directing arterial blood to the rele-vant venosome. Using this strategy, a 73% three year limb salvage rate was achieved [24].

7. Discussion

The concept of angiosome-directed revascularization is, theoretically, attractive and in ac-cordance with pathophysiological knowledge. It is also in line with experience from coro-nary bypass surgery, where reperfusion through collaterals does not provide a similar freedom from cardiac events as that provided by complete direct revascularization of all the diseased vascular territoria [2].

It is well established that healing of an ishemic pedal wound is more effectively ach-ieved when pulsatile arterial blood flow is established across the ankle and it seems logi-cal to expect that this effect is larger when the pulsatile flow is provided all the way to the site of the injury.

As suggested by the above mentioned papers, the effect of direct revascularization may es-pecially be relevant in the settings of end stage renal failure, infected wounds, endovascular rather than surgical repair, and in cases where collaterals are absent.

The angiosome concept represents a novel approach to improving the therapy of critical limb ischemia. It may potentially provide the rationale not only for the choice of target ar-tery. It may also influence the indications for endovascular or open repair according to which target artery is accessible by which method.

Although the evidence in favour of an angiosome directed treatment is mounting fast, it is, however, still circumstantial. All of the studies comparing the results of direct and indirect revascularization are retrospective and, thus, biased by heterogeneity in patient selection. More often than not, the angiosome specific artery will also be the most diseased artery and the ability to recanalize this vessel will most probably select the least atherosclerotic patients to the "direct revascularization" group. It is also likely that the advocates of an angiosome-directed revascularization strategy would attempt direct revascularization first and only perform indirect revascularization if this attempt was unsuccessful. Regardless of any retro-spective matching of the groups this would lead to patients with extensive distal atheroscle-rosis to be placed in the indirect revascularization groups, thus biasing the comparisons in favour of the angiosome specific approach. The differences in healing rate and limb salvage between groups may, therefore, merely reflect preoperative differences in the extent of oc-clusive disease. It is possible that this is what is reflected in the lack of statistically signifi-cant differences after propensity scoring in the study by Azuma [13].

As highlighted in the study by Varela, the presence or absence of collaterals merit further investigation [22]. For this purpose, the Doppler method described by Attinger [7] seems to be a good and non-invasive technique.

As evidence stands at the moment, there is some, although limited, evidence that when there is a choice of target artery for revascularization, preference should be given to the artery directly feeding the wound's angiosome. Specific analysis, based on prospectively collected data of homogeneous cohorts of patients are needed. Unbiased evidence will only be achievable by performing a prospective, randomized controlled trial with a blinded endpoint assessment.

Author details

Kim Houlind[1] and Johnny Christensen[2]

1 Dept. of Vascular Surgery, Kolding Hospital, Denmark and Institute of Regional Health Services Research, University of Southern Denmark, Denmark

2 Dept. of Radiology, Kolding Hospital, Denmark

References

[1] Norgreen L, Hiatt WR, Dormandy JA, Nehler MR, Harris KA, Fowkes FGR on behalf of the TASC II Working Group. Inter-society Concensus for the management of peripheral arterial disease (TASC II). Eur J Endovasc Surg 2007;33(Suppl 1): S32-55.

[2] Vieira RD, Hueb W, Gersh BJ, Lima EG, Pereira AC, Rezende PC, Garzillo CL, Hueb AC, Favarato D, Soares PR, Ramires JA, Filho RK. The effect of complete revascularization on 10-year Survival of Patients with Stable Multivessel Coronary artery Disease: MASS II Trial. Circulation 2012;126 (11 Suppl 1): S158-63

[3] Berceli SA, Chan AK, Pomposelli FB jr. Gibbons GW, Campbell DR, Akbari CM, Brophy DT, LoGerfo FW. Efficacy of dorsal pedal artery bypass in limb salvage for ischemic heel ulcers. J Vasc Surg 1999;30(3):499-508

[4] Taylor GI, Palmer JH. The vascular territories (angiosomes) of the body: Experimental study and clinical implication. Br J Plast Surg 1987;40:113-

[5] Taylor GI, Pan WR. Angiosomes of the leg: anatomic study and clinical implications. Plast Reconstr Surg 1998;102:599-616

[6] Clemens MW, Attinger CE. Angiosomes and wound care in the diabetic foot. Foot Ankle Clin N Am 2010;15:439-64

[7] Attinger CE, Evans KK, Bulan E, Blume P, Cooper P. Angiosomes of the Foot and Ankle and Clinical Implications for Limb Salvage: Reconstruction, Incisions, and Revascularization. Plast. Reconstr. Surg 2006; 117 (Suppl) 261S-293S

[8] Taylor GI, Corlett RJ, Caddy CM, Zelt RG. An anatomic review of the delay phenomenon: II. Clinical applications. Plast Reconstr Surg:89 (3):408-16

[9] Jörneskog G. Why critical limb ischemia criteria are not applicable to diabetic foot and what the consequences are. Scand J Surg 2012:101;114-18

[10] Manzi M, Cester G, Palena LM, Alek RT, Candeo A, Ferraresi R. Vascular Imaging of the Foot: The first step toward endovascular recanalization. Radiographics 2011;31(6):1623-36

[11] Nagase T, Sanada H, Takehara K, Oe M, Iizaka S, Ohashi Y, Oba M, Kadowaki T, Nakagami G. Variations of planatar thermographic patterns in normal controls and non-ulcer diabetic patients: Novel classification using angiosome concept. Journal of Plastic, reconstructive & aesthetic Surgery 2011; 64: 860-66

[12] Neville RF, attinger CE, Bulan EJ, Ducic I, Thomassen M, Sidaway AN. Revascularization of a Specific Angiosome for Limb salvage: Does the Target artery Matter? Ann Vasc Surg 2009;23:367-373

[13] Azuma N, Uchida H, kokubo T, Koya A, Akasaka N, sasajima T. factors influencing wound healing og critical ischaemic foot after bypass surgery: Is the angiosome important in selecting bypass traget artery. European journal of vascular and endovascular surgery 2012;43:322-328

[14] Iida O, Nanto S, Uematso M, Ikeoka K, Okamoto S, Dohi T, Fujita M, Terasi H, Nagata S. Importance of the angiosome concept for endovascular therapy in patients with critical limb ischemia. Catheterization and cardiovascular Interventions 2010; 75: 830-836

[15] Iida O, Soga Y, Hirano K, Kawasaki D, Suzuki K, Miyashita Y, Terasi H, Uematsu M. Long term reults of direct and indirect endovascular revascularization base don the angiosome concept in patients with critical limb ischemia presenting with isolated below-the knee lesions. J Vasc surg 2012;55:363-70

[16] Alexandriescu V-A, Hubermont G, Philips Y, Guillaumie B, Ngongang C, Vandenbossche P, Azdad K, Ledent G, Horion J. Selective primary angioplasty following an angiosome model of reperfusion in the treatment of Wagner 1-4 diabetic foot lesions: Practice in a multidisciplinary diabetic limb service. J Endovasc Ther 2008;15:580-593

[17] Alexandriescu V, Hubermont G. The challenging topic of diabetic foot revascularization: does the angiosome-guided angioplasty may improve outcome. Journal of Cardiovascular Surgery 2012;53:3-12.

[18] Alexandriescu V, Vincent G, Azdad K, Hubermont G, Ledent G, Ngongang C, Filimon A-M. A reliable approach to diabetic neuroischemic foot wounds: Below-the-knee angiosome-oriented angioplasty. J Endovasc Ther 2011;18:376-387

[19] Alexandriescu V, Söderström M, Venermo M. Angiosome theory: Fact or fiction? Scandinavian Journal of surgery 2012;101:125-31

[20] Deguchi J, Kitaoka T, Yamamoto K, Matsumoto H, Sato. Impact of Angiosome on Treatment of Diabetic Ischemic Foot with Paramalleolar Bypass. J Jpn Coll Angiol 2010;50:687-691

[21] Blanes Orti P, Vázquez R, Minguell P, García V, Manuel-Rimbau Munoz E, Lozarno Vilardell P. Percutaneous revascularization of specific angiosome in critical limb ischaemia. Angiologia 2011;63:11-17

[22] Varela C, Acin F, de Haro J, Bleda S, Esparza L, March JR. The role of foot collateral vessels on ulcer healing and limb salvage after successful endovascular and surgical distal procedures according to the angiosome model. Vasc Endovasc Surg 2010;44:654-660

[23] Taylor G.I, Caddy CM, Waterson PA, Crock JG. The venous territories (venosomes) of the human body. Experimental study and clinical implications. Plast Reconstr Surg 1990;86:185-

[24] Alexandriescu V, Ngongang C, Vincent G, Ledent G, Hubermont G. Deep calf veins arterialization for inferior limb preservation in diabetic patients with extended ischemic wounds, unfit for direct arterial reconstruction; preliminary results according to an angiosome model of perfusion. Cardiovascular revascularization Medicine 2011;12:10-19

Miscellaneous Cardiac Surgical Topics

Short and Long Term Effects of Psychosocial Factors on the Outcome of Coronary Artery Bypass Surgery

Zsuzsanna Cserép, Andrea Székely and Bela Merkely

Additional information is available at the end of the chapter

1. Introduction

Coronary heart disease (CHD) is the commonest form of heart disease in the developed world, and one of the leading causes of mortality and morbidity in these countries. Over the past decades numerous studies focused on the link between CHD and different psychosocial factors. The prevalence of depression in patients with diagnosed CHD is quoted between 20 and 45%. Elevated anxiety scores have been reported for 20 to 55% [1]. Emotional factors and the experience of chronic stress contribute to the development of atherosclerosis and cardiac events. Emotional factors include affective disorders such as major depression and anxiety disorders as well as hostility and anger. Chronic stressors include factors such as low social support and low socioeconomic status [2]. Similar prevalence ratios have been found for patients undergoing coronary artery bypass graft surgery (CABG). Symptoms of anxiety and unipolar depression are common psychological disturbances among patients undergoing CABG surgery. Numerous prospective cohort studies focus on the short and long term outcome of CABG. Research revealed that not only clinical factors e.g. cardiac status, comorbities and intraoperative factors have impact on the outcome [3]. Comparison of morbidity and mortality rates associated with psychosocial factors to morbidity and mortality rates related to traditional risk factors (smoking, obesity, and physical inactivity) showed priority of psychosocial background [4].

The purpose of this review is to provide a selected summary of key findings in this literature. We summarize some of the classic studies and historical developments important to the field and focus on prospective data on cardiac surgery patients. We review the literature on the important psychosocial domains (depression, anxiety, self rated health, happiness, illness intrusiveness, quality of life, gender differences, social support, negative affectivity, social inhibition, education) that have received much of the research attention, discuss key pathophysiological mechanisms and pathways by which psychosocial factors may influence the outcome after surgery, and discuss some treatment directions likely to be critical to advancing the field.

2. Depression

2.1. Depression and Coronary Heart Disease (CHD)

Among emotional factors, depression has been most widely studied in recent years. Depressive disorders vary from mild (subclinical) depressive symptoms to classic major depression. According to the Diagnostic and Statistical Manual of Mental Disorders, depression is characterized by low mood and/or anhedonia (lose interest in activities that once were pleasurable) that lasts for two weeks or more and is accompanied by significant functional impairment and somatic complaints (insomnia, excessive sleeping, fatigue, loss of energy, or aches, pains or digestive problems that are resistant to treatment) [2]. Depression is 3 times more common in patients after an acute myocardial infarction than in the general community. In-hospital prevalence of major depression was 15% to 20% of patients with myocardial infarction, and an even more patients showed an elevated level of depressive symptoms [5]. Depression is regarded as an independent risk factor for atherosclerotic deposits in coronary arteries. The pathophysiological background covers hypercortisolaemia related to e.g. insulin resistance, sympathetic vagal dysbalance related to e.g. disturbed regulation of blood pressure, reduced heart rate variability, hypothalamic-pituitary-adrenal axis dysfunction, increased plasma platelet factor 4 (suggesting enhanced platelet activation), impaired vascular function, and increased C-reactive protein and fibrinogen levels (suggesting increased inflammatory response) and an unfavourable lifestyle like cigarette smoking, unhealthy diet, and lack of physical activity, medication adherence, as well as social isolation and chronic life stress [1, 5]. Depressive patients have higher risk of non-compliance with medical treatment regimens, therefore reduced chances of successful modifications of other cardiac risk factors and participation in cardiac rehabilitation, and have greatly reduced quality of life [5]. Major depression and elevated depressive symptoms are associated with worse prognosis in patients with CHD: in the Prospective Epidemiological Study of Myocardial Infarction (PRIME) Study, a multicenter, observational, prospective cohort, in healthy, European, middle-aged men were surveyed for the occurrence of first coronary heart disease and stroke events over 10 years. At baseline a questionnaire was used to define the presence of depressive symptoms. Results suggested that, baseline depressive symptoms are associated with an increased risk of coronary heart disease in the short-term and for stroke in the long-term [6]. Barefoot et al. assessed 1250 patients with documented CHD using the Zung Self-Report Depression Scale at the time of diagnostic coronary angiography and followed patients for up to 19.4 years. Results showed that patients with moderate to severe depression were at 69% greater risk for cardiac death and 78% greater risk for all-cause death [7]. Frasure-Smith et al. assessed gender differences in the impact of depression on 1-year cardiac mortality in patients hospitalized for an acute myocardial infarction. Increased depression scores were significantly related to cardiac mortality for both genders (the odds ratio for women was 3.29, for men, the odds ratio was 3.05). Data were controlled for other multivariate predictors of mortality (age, Killip class, the interactions of gender by non-Q wave myocardial infarction, gender by left ventricular ejection fraction, and gender by smoking) and showed that depression was independent predictor for either gender [8]. Most studies that have examined the relationship between increasing depression severity and cardiac events have shown a dose-response relationship: in a 5-year-follow-up study post-myocardial infarction patients were recruited and assigned to categories based on the severity of depressive symptoms, ranging from no depressive symptoms to moderate to severe depressive symptoms. During follow-up period, a gradient relationship was observed between the magnitude of depressive symptoms and the frequency of deaths, with increased events occurring even in patients with mild depressive symptoms [9]. In the prospective study of Brown et al. elderly adults with significant depressive symptoms at baseline and without a current diagnosis of CHD at baseline were more likely to experience a cardiac event over a 15-year follow-up period. Depressed patients were 1.5 times more likely to suffer a cardiac event (i.e., acute myocardial infarction or cardiac death), even after controlling for demographics and known cardiovascular risk factors. The elevated depressive symptom severity is a predictor of cardiac events among older women and men as well as older white and black adults [10]. Despite methodological differences (sample sizes, sample characteristics, selection of covariates, etc) from study to study, the data from prospective studies with objective outcome measures and validated question-naires for depression are remarkably consistent in their results suggesting depression is a risk factor for both the development of and the worsening of CHD [5].

2.2. Depression and CABG

CABG surgery is a common surgical intervention for CHD patients and prevalence of depression before or after CABG surgery is about 20–25% [4]. The presence of elevated levels of depressive symptoms results in a higher risk of mortality and significantly increased overall risk of major cardiac events following cardiac surgery [11]. In the prospective study of Connerney et al. 309 CABG patients were followed for 1 year after surgery. Compared with non depressed patients, depressed patients were more than twice as likely to have a cardiac event within 12 months after surgery but were not at higher risk for mortality within the first year [4]. In a larger sample of 817 CABG patients followed for up to 12 years, Blumenthal et al. assessed the effect of depression on mortality after CABG surgery. Depression was assessed both at baseline and 6 months after surgery. Results indicated that moderate to severe depression on the day before surgery as well as depression that persisted from baseline to 6 months after surgery were associated with 2-fold to 3-fold increased risk of mortality after adjustment for other risk factors [3]. Readmission following cardiac surgery is a significant burden on the healthcare system. In a prospective study, 226 CABG patients completed baseline self-report measures of depression, anxiety and stress and 222 patients completed these measures after surgery on the hospital ward. In multivariable analyses more than two-fold increase in readmission risk was associated with preoperative anxiety and postoperative depression, independent of covariates [12]. When our work group investigated the relationship between depression, anxiety, education, social isolation and mortality 7.5 years after cardiac surgery, we found that there was a significant difference in depression (measured with Beck Depression Inventory (BDI)) between survivors and non survivors preoperatively, after discharge and in both intervals (Figure 1) [13].

First author and title	Number of patients	Methods	Results
Blumenthal JA. Depression as a risk factor for mortality after coronary artery bypass surgery.	817	CABG patients completed the Center for Epidemiological Studies-Depression (CES-D) scale before surgery, 6 months after CABG, and were followed-up for up to 12 years.	Patients with moderate to severe depression at baseline (adjusted hazard ratio [HR] 2.4, [95% CI 1.4-4.0]; p=0.001) and mild or moderate to severe depression that persisted from baseline to 6 months (adjusted HR 2.2, [1.2-4.2]; p=0.015) had higher rates of death than did those with no depression
Connerney I. Relation between depression after coronary artery bypass surgery and 12-month outcome: a prospective study.	207 men and 102 women	CABG patients screened for depression with a structured psychiatric interview (diagnostic interview schedule) and a questionnaire (Beck depression inventory) before discharge. Outcome: cardiac events included angina or heart failure that needed admission to hospital, myocardial infarction, cardiac arrest, percutaneous transluminal coronary angioplasty, repeat CABG, and cardiac mortality. Non-cardiac events consisted of all other reasons for mortality or readmission.	63 patients (20%) met criteria for major depressive disorder. At 12 months, 17 (27%) of these patients had a cardiac event compared with 25 of 246 (10%) who were not depressed (p<0.0008). In a Cox proportional-hazard model with these five and two other variables of cardiac severity, major depressive disorder (risk ratio 2.3 [95% CI 1.17-4.56]), low ejection fraction (2.3 [1.07-5.03]), and female sex (2.4 [1.24-4.44]) were associated with adverse outcomes. Depression did not predict deaths or admissions for non-cardiac events.
Majed B. Depressive symptoms, a time-dependent risk factor for coronary heart disease and stroke in middle-aged men: the PRIME Study.	9601 men	The occurrence of first coronary heart disease (n=647) and stroke events (n=136) over 10 years among healthy men.	Depressive symptoms at baseline were associated with coronary heart disease in the first 5 years of follow-up (hazard ratio, 1.43, 1.10-1.87) and with stroke in the second 5 years of follow up (hazard ratio, 1.96; 1.21-3.19) after adjustment. The association was even stronger for ischemic stroke (n=108; hazard ratio, 2.48; 1.45-4.25).
Barefoot JC. Depression and long-term mortality risk in patients with coronary artery disease.	1250	Patients with established CAD were assessed for depression with the Zung Self-Rating Depression Scale and followed for subsequent mortality. Follow-up ranged up to 19.4 years.	Depression was associated with increased risk of cardiac death (p = 0.002) and total mortality (p < 0.001) after controlling for initial disease severity and treatment. Patients with moderate to severe depression had a 69% greater odds of cardiac death and a 78% greater odds of mortality from all causes than nondepressed patients. Patients with moderate to severe

			depression had an 84% greater risk 5 to 10 years later and a 72% greater risk after "/> 10 years compared with the nondepressed.
Frasure-Smith N. Gender, depression, and one-year prognosis after myocardial infarction.	613 men 283 women	Beck Depression Inventory (BDI) was used to assess depression symptoms during hospitalization after an acute myocardial infarction.	There were 290 patients (133 women) with at least mild to moderate symptoms of depression; 8.3% of the depressed women died of cardiac causes in contrast to 2.7% of the nondepressed. For depressed men, the rate of cardiac death was 7.0% in contrast to 2.4% of the nondepressed. Increased BDI scores were significantly related to cardiac mortality for both genders [the odds ratio for women was 3.29 (95% confidence interval (CI) = 1.02-10.59); for men, the odds ratio was 3.05 (95% CI = 1.29-7.17)]. Control for other multivariate predictors of mortality in the data set (age, Killip class, the interactions of gender by non-Q wave MI, gender by left ventricular ejection fraction, and gender by smoking) did not change the impact of the BDI for either gender.
Lesperance F. Five-year risk of cardiac mortality in relation to initial severity and one-year changes in depression symptoms after myocardial infarction	896	Beck Depression Inventory was administered to the patients after myocardial infarction during admission and at 1 year. Five-year survival was ascertained using Medicare data	Significant long-term dose-response relationship between depression symptoms during hospitalization and cardiac mortality was observed. Results remained significant after control for multiple measures of cardiac disease severity. Although 1-year scores were also linked to cardiac mortality, most of that impact was explained by baseline scores. Improvement in depression symptoms was associated with less cardiac mortality only for patients with mild depression. Patients with higher initial scores had worse long-term prognosis regardless of symptom changes.
Brown JM. Risk of coronary heart disease events over 15 years among older adults with depressive symptoms	2728	Depressive symptom severity at baseline was assessed by the Center for Epidemiologic Studies Depression Scale among primary care practice patients. Data regarding baseline demographic and clinical variables, as well as laboratory evidence of acute MI, were obtained from an electronic medical record system. All-cause mortality and CHD death were determined from the National Death Index through 2006.	Cox proportional hazards models showed that individuals with elevated depressive symptoms were more likely to experience a CHD event, even after adjustment for demographics and comorbid health conditions (relative risk = 1.46, 95% confidence interval: 1.20-1.77). Depression status was also a significant predictor of all-cause mortality in adjusted models.

| Tully PJ. The role of depression and anxiety symptoms in hospital readmissions after cardiac surgery. | 226 | Hospital readmissions after coronary artery bypass graft surgery were assessed. | When analyzed as continuous variables in multivariable analyses, preoperative anxiety and postoperative depression predicted readmissions independent of medical covariates. In multivariable analyses with dichotomized anxiety, depression and stress, more than two-fold increase in readmission risk was attributable to preoperative anxiety and postoperative depression, independent of covariates. |

Table 1. Some important studies about depression and CABG

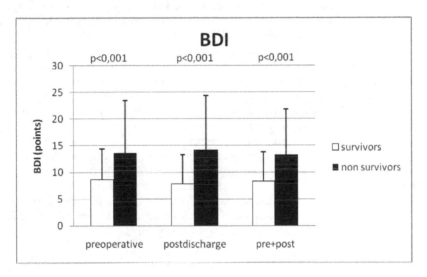

Figure 1. Figure showes significant difference in depression (BDI points) between survivors and non survivors preoperatively, after discharge and in both intervals.

3. Anxiety

3.1. Anxiety and coronary heart disease

Anxiety has been characterized as a future-oriented, negative affective state with a component of fear, resulting from the perception of threat and the individual's perceived inability to predict, control, or obtain the desired results in upcoming situations. Somatic manifestations are tachycardia, hyperventilation, sweating, psychological manifestations are feelings of apprehension, nervousness, restlessness, and may also cause changes in sleeping pattern [13].

Pathophysiological background by which anxiety influences outcome in ischemic heart disease is largely unknown. An increased incidence of ECG QT interval prolongation has been demonstrated among patients with anxiety, which increases the occurrence of ventricular arrhythmia [14]. Patients with anxiety have been shown consistently to have sympathetic nervous system upregulation, with excessive catecholamine production [15]. Furthermore, impaired vagal control, manifest as an impaired baroreflex response and a decrease in heart rate variability has been noted in patients with anxiety. Impairment of the baroreflex response and decreased heart rate variability are each thought to be sensitive markers for abnormalities in autonomic cardiovascular regulation and are independent risk factors for sudden cardiac death [16, 17, 18]. Patients with anxiety and CAD often show an exaggerated systemic response to stress, characterized by an abnormally increased production of catecholamines, which can result in increased myocardial oxygen demand due to elevations in heart rate, blood pressure, and the rate of ventricular contraction [19]. In addition to the biological risks of anxiety, the additive effects of adverse behavioural risk factors (e.g., excessive nicotine and perhaps caffeine) in anxious patients have also be taken into account [20]. Anxiety is very common in patients with myocardial infarction, with an inhospital occurrence rate of 30% to 40% [21]. Studies with coronary patients suggest that anxiety disorders may be associated with greater mortality, particularly sudden cardiac death, and greater cardiovascular morbidity. Higher levels of anxiety have been associated with poorer prognosis and greater recurrence of cardiac events after myocardial infarction [22]. In a cohort study the relative importance of depression, anxiety, anger, and social support in predicting 5-year cardiac-related mortality following a myocardial infarction was investigated. Higher level of anxiety predicted greater cardiac-related mortality in a sample of nearly 900 patients with myocardial infarction, but this effect was non significant following adjustment for disease severity [23]. The first meta-analysis on the association of anxiety and coronary heart disease showed a consistent association between anxiety and impaired prognosis after myocardial infarction, with a 36% increased risk for mortality (cardiac and all-cause) and for cardiac events. Limitation of the result was the pooled odds ratios for cardiac death, because it was based on only four studies [21].

3.2. Anxiety and CABG

Anxiety is especially high for CABG patients while they are on the waiting list with an unknown surgery date [24]. The patients have fear of dying before, rather than during surgery, and this fear influenced strongly their level of anxiety. Anxiety also manifests as an activator of sympathetic and parasympathetic nervous systems and cardiovascular excitation that can exacerbate CAD symptoms. After surgery, while anxiety may decrease to below pre-operative level, the severity of anxiety does not necessarily remit to below sub-clinical levels and may warrant intervention [25]. In the Post-CABG Trial the presence of anxiety symptoms was significantly associated with a higher incidence rate of death or myocardial infarction after a median follow-up time of 4.3 years following CABG. After controlling for the presence of depressive symptoms and other covariates (age, gender, race, treatment assignment and years since CABG surgery), a significant dose-response relationship persisted between anxiety and mortality. The observed dose-response relationship between level of anxiety and risk of death or myocardial infarction underlines the importance of even lower levels of anxiety. The risk of death or myocardial infarction in those with both depressive and anxiety symptoms was what would be expected from the combination of the independent effects [26]. In a study of our workgroup trait anxiety was associated with increased mortality and cardiovascular morbidity. In our population trait anxiety remained an independent predictor for post-discharge cardiovascular events and 4 year mortality. Moreover, post-discharge 6th month trait anxiety scores were more predictive for cardiovascular events compared to the preoperative values. Although anxiety and depression were positively and highly correlated in these patients, only anxiety was associated with increased mortality and morbidity. In addition trait anxiety was significantly higher in patients hospitalized with arrhythmia, congestive heart failure or myocardial infarction during a 4 year period after cardiac (CABG and valve) surgery [27]. In another study of our workgroup depression, anxiety, education, social isolation and mortality together were investigated 7.5 years after cardiac surgery. Our results have suggested that the assessment of psychosocial factors, particularly anxiety and education may help identify patients at an increased risk for long-term mortality after cardiac surgery (Figure 2.) [13]. Anxiety was also reported to be associated with twofold risk for fatal CHD and more than fourfold risk for sudden death [28]. In a retrospective study 17,885 discharge records of patients after primary CABG surgery were identified. In the sample of rural patients the prevalence of anxiety disorder was 27%. Anxiety was a significant independent predictor of both length of hospital stay and non routine discharge [29]. In a prospective study on cardiac-related readmission within 6 months of CABG postoperative anxiety was identified as both a univariate risk factor and a multivariate risk factor for CHD and surgery-related readmission both with and without adjustment for covariates [30].

First author and title	Number of patients	Methods	Results
Cserep Z. The impact of preoperative anxiety and education level on long-term mortality after cardiac surgery.	180	Anxiety (Spielberger State-Trait Anxiety Inventory, STAI-S/STAI-T), depression (Beck Depression Inventory, BDI) and the number and reason for rehospitalizations were assessed each year in cardiac surgery patients.	During a median follow-up of 7.6 years (25th to 75th percentile, 7.4 to 8.1 years), the mortality rate was 23.6% (95% confidence Interval [CI] 17.3-29.9; 42 deaths). In a Cox regression model, the risk factors associated with an increased risk of mortality were a higher EUROSCORE (points; Adjusted Hazard Ratio (AHR):1.30, 95%CI:1.07-1.58)), a higher preoperative STAI-T score (points; AHR:1.06, 95%CI 1.02-1.09), lower education level (school years; AHR:0.86, 95%CI:0.74-0.98), and the occurrence of major adverse cardiac and cerebral events during follow up (AHR:7.24, 95%CI: 2.65-19.7). In the postdischarge model, the same risk factors remained.

Frasure-Smith N. Depression and other psychological risks following myocardial infarction	896	Beck Depression Inventory, state scale of the State-Trait Anxiety Inventory, 20-item version of the General Health Questionnaire, Modified Somatic Perception Questionnaire, Anger Expression Scale, Perceived Social Support Scale, number of close friends and relatives, and visual analog scales of anger and stress were assessed to predict 5-year cardiac-related mortality following a myocardial infarction.	The Beck Depression Inventory (P<0.001), the State-Trait Anxiety Inventory (P =0.04), and the 20-item version of the General Health Questionnaire (P = 0.048) were related to outcome, but only depression remained significant after adjustment for cardiac disease severity (hazards ratio per SD, 1.46; 95% confidence interval, 1.18-1.79) (P<0.001). There was also a covariate-adjusted trend between negative affectivity scores and outcome (P = 0.08). Furthermore, residual depression scores (P =0.001) and negative affectivity scores (P = 0.05) were linked to cardiac-related mortality after adjustment for each other and cardiac covariates.
Koivula M. Fear and anxiety in patients at different time-points in the coronary artery bypass process.	171	CABG patients completed questionnaires while awaiting surgery at home, in hospital the evening before surgery and 3 months later. The Bypass Grafting Fear scale was developed to measure fear. Anxiety was measured using State-Trait-Anxiety Inventory.	The highest levels of fear and anxiety were measured in the waiting period to coronary CABG. Compared with the waiting period, fear and anxiety levels dropped in hospital and 3 months later. Female gender was related to change in fear and anxiety.
Rosenbloom JI. Self-reported anxiety and the risk of clinical events and atherosclerotic progression among patients with Coronary Artery Bypass Grafts (CABG).	1317	CABG patients were randomized to either aggressive or moderate lipid lowering and to either warfarin or placebo. Patients were followed up for clinical end points and coronary angiography was conducted at enrollment and after a median follow-up of 4.3 years. Anxiety symptoms were assessed at enrollment using the state portion of the Spielberger State-Trait Anxiety Inventory (STAI)	STAI score "/> or =40 was positively associated with risk of death or myocardial infarction (MI) (OR 1.55, 95% CI 1.01-2.36, P =0.044). This association was attenuated slightly when depressive symptoms were included in the model, but lost statistical significance (P = 0.11). There was a dose-response relationship between STAI score and risk of death or myocardial infarction. There was no association between self-reported anxiety and atherosclerotic progression of grafts.
Székely A. Anxiety predicts mortality and morbidity after coronary artery and valve surgery--a 4-year follow-up study.	180	Patients who underwent cardiac surgery using cardiopulmonary bypass were prospectively studied and followed up for 4 years. Anxiety (Spielberger State-Trait Anxiety Inventory, STAI-S/STAI-T), depression (Beck Depression Inventory, BDI), living alone, and education level along with clinical risk factors and	Average preoperative STAI-T score was 44.6 +/- 10. Kaplan-Meier analysis showed a significant effect of preoperative STAI-T "/>45 points (p =0.008) on mortality. In multivariate models, postoperative congestive heart failure (OR: 10.8; 95% confidence interval [CI]: 2.9-40.1; p =0 .009) and preoperative

		perioperative characteristics were assessed. Psychological self-report questionnaires were completed preoperatively and 6, 12, 24, 36, and 48 months after discharge. Clinical endpoints were mortality and cardiac events requiring hospitalization during follow-up.	STAI-T (score OR: 1.07; 95% CI: 1.01-1.15; p = 0.05) were independently associated with mortality. The occurrence of cardiovascular hospitalization was independently associated with postoperative intensive care unit days (OR: 1.41; 95% CI: 1.01-1.96; p =0.045) and post discharge 6th month STAI-T (OR: 1.06; 95% CI:1.01-1.13; p = .03).
Kawachi I. Symptoms of anxiety and risk of coronary heart disease. The Normative Aging Study.	402 cases of incident coronary heart disease	An anxiety symptoms scale was constructed out of five items from the Cornell Medical Index, which was administered to the cohort at baseline. During 32 years of follow-up incidence of CHD was observed.	Compared with men reporting no symptoms of anxiety, men reporting two or more anxiety symptoms had elevated risks of fatal CHD (age-adjusted odds ratio [OR] = 3.20, 95% confidence interval [CI]: 1.27 to 8.09), and sudden death (age-adjusted OR = 5.73, 95% CI: 1.26 to 26.1). The multivariate OR after adjusting for a range of potential confounding variables was 1.94 (95% CI: 0.70-5.41) for fatal CHD and 4.46 (95% CI: 0.92-21.6) for sudden death. No excess risks were found for nonfatal myocardial infarction or angina.
Dao TK. Gender as a moderator between having an anxiety disorder diagnosis and coronary artery bypass grafting surgery (CABG) outcomes in rural patients.	17,885	Patients who underwent a primary CABG surgery were identified. Independent variables included age, gender, race, median household income based on patient's ZIP code, primary expected payer, the Deyo, Cherkin, and Ciol Comorbidity Index, and an anxiety comorbidity diagnosis. Outcome variables included in-hospital length of stay and patient disposition (routine and nonroutine discharge).	27% of rural patients had a comorbid anxiety diagnosis. Rural patients who had nonroutine discharge were more likely to have comorbid anxiety diagnosis compared to rural patients who had a routine discharge. There was a significant interaction effect between having an anxiety diagnosis and gender on length of hospital stay but not for patient disposition.
Oxlad M. Psychological risk factors for cardiac-related hospital readmission within 6 months of coronary artery bypass graft surgery.	119	Consecutive patients awaiting elective CABG, completed a battery of psychosocial measures in a three-stage repeated-measures design. Relevant medical data were also extracted from patients' medical records 6 months postoperatively to allow for the examination of potential covariates.	Increased postoperative anxiety and increased preoperative depression, were identified as risk factors for cardiac-related readmission independent of the only significant covariate identified, cardiopulmonary bypass time.

Table 2. Some important studies about anxiety and CABG

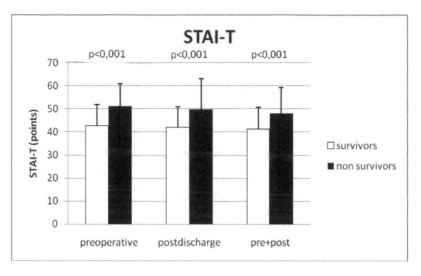

Figure 2. Figure showes significant difference in STAI-T (State-Trait Anxiety Inventory) between survivors and non survivors preoperatively, after discharge and in both intervals.

4. Self rated health

Self-rated health (SRH) is measured with a simple question "How do you rate your health in general?" There are five possible responses: very good, good, fair, poor and very poor [31]. Self rated health has been shown to be a potent predictor of mortality and morbidity, functional decline, disability and utilization of health care even after controlling for several sociodemographic and health indicators The association can be explained by three ways: (1) SRH is a more comprehensive and sensitive measure of health status than the other psychosocial covariates in the analyses; (2) SRH measures individual optimistic or pessimistic disposition, that as such, may be associated with survival; or (3) SRH also measures characteristics other than health status itself, such as family history, health behaviour, and social and psychological resources [32]. In a review SRH was described as an active cognitive process that is independent from formal definitions of health. Self rated health covers bodily sensations that are directly available only to the individuals. These sensations may reflect important physiological dysregulations, such as inflammatory processes. SRH is an individual and subjective conception that is related to death, and builds a connection from the social world and psychological to the biological world. Therefore the answer to the SRH question may summarize the dimensions of health that are most important and determinant to each individual [33]. SRH has been described as one of the most important health outcomes available and recommended as a tool for disease risk screening, as an outcome indicator in the primary care, and standard part of clinical trials [34]. Several studies in different field confirmed the importance of SRH, one of them described that good self health 3 months after PCI predicted good clinical outcome after 4 years [35]. SRH was reported as an independent predictor of long term mortality in older women after myocardial infarction. Patients dissatisfied with their general health status were at more than six times higher risk of mortality than the satisfied ones [36]. There are only few data available on the link between CABG and SRH. Oxlad et al. investigated consecutive elective CABG patients on self-report measures including optimism, illness representations, self-rated health, social support, coping methods, depression, anxiety and post-traumatic stress disorder. Poor pre-operative psychological functioning was the strongest psychological risk factor for adverse psychological functioning six months post-operatively [37].

5. Happiness

Negative emotional states (e.g., depression, anxiety) are proven risk factors for cardiovascular disease; however, much less is known about the association between positive emotional states (e.g., happiness and optimism) and cardiovascular health. Steptoe et al. have suggested that positive emotions may have direct and beneficial effects on physiological processes including those involving the neuroendocrine, inflammatory, immunological and cardiovascular systems [38]. The association between positive psychological well-being and mortality could be mediated in part via behavioural pathways. For example positive dispositions are related to predictors of prolonged survival, such as not smoking, exercising regularly, reduced alcohol consumption, and better sleep quality. Psychologically balanced persons might have increased adherence to medical regimens because inverse associations between adherence and depression have been described. However, the protective effect of positive emotions on mortality in healthy population studies persisted even after fully controlling for behavioural covariates, suggesting that other pathways may also be involved. Direct physiological pathways might also contribute to associations. Positive psychological well-being could alter people's disease susceptibility via the attenuation of sympathetic nervous system activity and the enhancement of parasympathetic activation. Positive affects may reduce stress-induced elevations of inflammatory and coagulation factors, such as fibrinogen and interleukin-6, which are crucial in cardiovascular disease, and reduce vulnerability to infectious illness. Positive psychological well-being was associated with reduced cardiovascular mortality in healthy population studies, with a near significant effect in patients with established cardiovascular disease [39]. In one of prospective epidemiological cohort studies participants with greater emotional vitality were at markedly reduced risk for CHD, and this effect remained significant after controlling for medical and psychosocial factors [40]. Optimism was associated with recovery from CABG surgery within 6 months [41]. Post hoc analysis of previous data showed that among depressed post-CABG patients, optimists responded to depression treatment at higher rates. Independent of depression, optimists were less likely to be rehospitalized by 8 months after CABG [42].

6. Illness intrusiveness

One of the important determinants of quality of life is taking part in psychologically meaningful activity. Illnesses, mostly chronic ones interfere with valued activities. Illness intrusiveness is a determinant of quality of life in patients with chronic disease. Illness intrusiveness covers the disease- and treatment-induced disruptions to lifestyles, activities, and interests [43]. There is only one available study about the relationship of illness intrusiveness and CABG: our work group investigated psychosocial factors like illness intrusiveness, depression, anxiety, sleeping disorders and found an independent association with the occurrence of major adverse cardiac and cerebrovascular events (MACCE) after adjustment of biomedical factors and perioperative variables following cardiac surgery. Additionally, severity of illness intrusiveness, sleeping problems and social inhibition increased in the MACCE positive patients during the three-year period; these tendencies were not observed in the event-free group [44].

7. Quality of life

With aging of the population and sophisticated health care technologies the number of patients with chronic diseases has extremely increased. As a result, improving the daily functioning and quality of life of the chronically ill has become an important goal of medical and surgical interventions. Therefore assessing the quality of life has been brought into the limelight [45]. On the other hand, predictive value of quality of life on survival and other outcomes of cardiac surgery has been also studied. In a prospective study of 6305 patients who underwent isolated coronary artery bypass the overall functional health-related quality of life improved after recovery from cardiac surgery. Reduced long-term survival following cardiac surgery even after adjustment for known risk factors associated with survival after cardiac surgery was associated with lower functional health related quality of life beyond the posthospital recovery phase. The degree of functional recovery was directly related to subsequent survival [46]. In a prospective cohort study the preoperative quality of life was an independent predictor of 6-month mortality following CABG even after adjusting for traditional risk factors. The magnitude of the effect (39% increase in risk for a small difference in quality of life score) was clinically important, and it is a non-invasive, easily available tool for clinicians [47].

8. Gender differences

The increased operative mortality and morbidity of women compared with men undergoing CABG surgery results from differences in methodology, low number of women in studies reporting negative findings, many studies, both positive and negative, did not take into account preoperative differences in health status between the sexes. Women more frequently have factors associated with increased short- and long-term mortality, such as less common use of internal mammary artery grafts. According to the reported analyses, they are older, less educated, have more severe angina and congestive heart failure, lower functional status, and higher level of depressive symptoms. At time of referral, women are at more advanced disease stage than men; however, despite being more symptomatic, women have less extensive coronary artery disease than men as determined by coronary angiography results [48]. This large number of differences makes the comparison difficult, and studies are not corrected for so many potential imbalances that may influence sex differences in outcome. Additional large prospective studies with substantial numbers of women are needed to evaluate gender-related differences in autonomic responses to myocardial infarction, complications related to cardio-pulmonary bypass, susceptibility to abnormalities in coagulation, and other biological factors that might account for discrepant outcomes in men versus women undergoing CABG. Furthermore, specific pharmacologic and therapeutic considerations, such as the role of estrogen replacement therapy, need to be clarified [49]. Compared to conducted studies in this topic the POST CABG Biobehavioral Study enrolled the highest number of women (n = 269) and physical, social, and emotional functioning were investigated after CABG surgery. Both male and female patients improved in physical, social, and emotional functioning after CABG, and recovery over time was similar in men and women. However, women's health-related quality-of-life scale scores remained less favourable than men's women did show less benefit with regard to the symptoms of shortness of breath and tiredness through 1 year after surgery [50]. In another prospective cohort study on quality of life women did not reach the same degree of improvement after 1 year as men, even after adjusting for pre-existing risk factors. Women were at greater risk for subjective cognitive difficulties, increased anxiety and decreased ability to perform tasks for daily living, diminished work-related activities, and reduced exercise capacity [51].

9. Social support

Socially isolated persons are single and/or have small social network. Social isolation is associated with poor outcome in established CAD, while high levels of social support is known to promote psychologic and physical well being [52]. Social support can be divided into two broad categories: social networks, which describe the size, structure, and frequency of contact with the network of people surrounding an individual; and functional support, which may be further divided into received social support, which highlights the type and amount of resources provided by the social network, and perceived social support, which focuses on the subjective satisfaction with available support or the perception that support would be available if needed [2]. The underlying mechanisms remain to be identified. Several factors may confound the effect of isolation such as disease severity, or its associations with demographic measures, because socially isolated patients are generally older and of lower socioeconomic status, which are known to reduce survival. Another possible mechanism is the influence of disease progression via its effect on psychosocial functioning. Psychological distress in CAD patients is more severe in patients with lack of adequate social support. Description of the demographic and psychosocial characteristics of those with few social contacts might aid our understanding of the link between isolation and mortality [52]. Previous studies showed the pivotal role of family ties in preserving cardiovascular health [53, 54]. A strong and consistent inverse gradient was reported between the magnitude of social support and adverse clinical outcomes among both initially healthy subjects and those with known CAD [55]. In our study on cardiac surgery patients (180 patients) 17% of patients admitted living alone, however when asking about marital status 35% admitted being single. We showed in our study that social isolation was associated with higher mortality after cardiac surgery [27]. Without social network and family support patients face longer hospital stay after CABG. Loneliness increases mortality: in a prospective study 1290 CABG patients were investigated. After controlling for various preoperative factors known to be independently associated with mortality loneliness was found to be associated with mortality, both at 30 days (relative risk 2.61) and at 5 years (relative risk 1.78) after the operation [52]. Kopp et al. found that marital status and spouse support was closely associated with men's mortality. Premature death was significantly lower among married men or men in relationship compared to single men and those who were satisfied with spouse support compared to those who were not [56]. Orth-Gomer et al. reported that following myocardial infarction, women with concomitant marital stress had 2.9-fold increased risk of recurrent cardiac events during a five-year follow-up compared to those with less marital stress after adjustment for age, estrogen status, education level, smoking, diagnosis at index event, diabetes mellitus, systolic blood pressure, smoking, triglyceride level, high-density lipoprotein cholesterol level, and left ventricular dysfunction [57]. In accordance with this finding, higher prevalence of subclinical atherosclerosis, and accelerated progression over time, among healthy women reporting marital dissatisfaction was reported, assuming that marital stress is atherogenic [58].

10. Negative affectivity and social inhibition

Type D personality unifies psychosocial factors related to high cardiovascular risk in one model. Particularly negative affectivity (NA) and social inhibition (SI) are relevant in this context. NA refers to the stable tendency to experience negative emotions across time/ situations. Persons with high-NA experience more feelings of dysphoria, anxiety, and irritability; have a negative view of self; and are looking for signs of impending trouble. NA overlaps with neuroticism and trait anxiety; includes subjective feelings of tension, worry, anxiety, anger, and sadness. SI patients tend to inhibit the expression of emotions/behaviours in social interactions to avoid disapproval by others. They feel inhibited, tense, and insecure when with others. Individuals who are high in both NA and SI have a distressed or Type D personality, given their vulnerability to chronic distress [59]. Type D patients are at increased risk for a wide range of adverse health outcomes, mortality and morbidity, in various cardio-vascular populations, including those with ischemic heart disease [60], coronary intervention [61], cardiac arrhythmias [62], peripheral arterial disease [63]. Global left ventricular dysfunc-tion and type D personality were independent predictors of long-term cardiac events in patients with a reduced ejection fraction after myocardial infarction [64]. Type D personality independently predicted mortality and early allograft rejection after heart transplantation [65]. In our 5-year follow-up, there was no link between the occurrence of major cardiac and cerebral event and NA and SI after CABG [44]. Additionally, severity of illness intrusiveness, sleeping problems and SI increased in the MACCE positive patients during the three-year period Unfavourable effect of Type D is linked to physiological hyperreactivity, immune activation, and inadequate response to cardiac treatment [59].

First author and title	Number of patients	Methods	Results
Cserép Z. Psychosocial factors and major adverse cardiac and cerebrovascular events after cardiac surgery.	180	Depression [Beck depression inventory (BDI)], anxiety [state anxiety subscale in Spielberger State-Trait Anxiety Inventory (STAI-S) and trait anxiety subscale in Spielberger State-Trait Anxiety Inventory (STAI-T)] were investigated annually, social support, negative affectivity, social inhibition (SI), illness intrusiveness, self-rated health and sleeping disorders were investigated by standardized tests at the second and fifth year after cardiac surgery. The end-point was the major adverse cardiac and cerebrovascular event (MACCE) including death.	At the end of the second year after adjustment for medical and perioperative factors worse self-rated health [adjusted hazard ratio (AHR): 0.67, P=0.006], sleeping disorders (AHR: 1.14, P=0.001), higher illness intrusiveness (AHR: 1.03, P=0.018), higher BDI (AHR: 1.12, P=0.001), STAI-S (AHR: 1.09, P=0.001) and higher STAI T scores (AHR: 1.08, P=0.002) showed higher risk for MACCE. Significant individual elevation in scores of sleeping disorders, illness intrusiveness and SI were observed over the three-year period in the MACCE group.
Denollet J. Personality as independent predictor of long-term mortality in patients with coronary heart disease.	268 men and 35 women	Patients with angiographically documented CHD, who were taking part in an outpatient rehabilitation programme. All patients completed personality questionnaire at entry to the programme. Survival status was followed up for mean 7-9 years. The main endpoint was death from all causes.	The rate of death was higher for type-D patients than for those without type-D (23 [27%]/85 vs 15 [7%]/218; p < 0.00001). The association between type-D personality and mortality was still evident more than 5 years after the coronary event and was found in both men and women. Type-D was an independent predictor of both cardiac and non-cardiac mortality after controlling for medial variables.
Pedersen SS. Type D personality predicts death or myocardial infarction after bare metal stent or sirolimus-eluting stent implantation: a Rapamycin-Eluting Stent Evaluated At Rotterdam Cardiology Hospital (RESEARCH) registry sub-study.	875	Patients completed the Type D Personality Scale (DS14) six months after PCI. The end point was a composite of death and MI.	Type D patients were at a cumulative increased risk of adverse outcome compared with non-Type D patients: 5.6% versus 1.3% (p < 0.002). Type D personality (odds ratio [OR] 5.31; 95% confidence interval [CI] 2.06 to 13.66) remained an independent predictor of adverse outcome adjusting for all other variables.

Pedersen SS. Type D personality is associated with increased anxiety and depressive symptoms in patients with an implantable cardioverter defibrillator and their partners.	221	Patients with implantable cardioverter defibrillator and their partners completed the Hospital Anxiety and Depression Scale, the Type D Personality Scale, and the Perceived Social Support Scale.	In patients, Type D personality was independently related to anxiety (OR: 7.03; 95% CI: 2.32-21.32) and depressive symptoms (OR: 7.40; 95% CI: 2.49-21.94) adjusting for all other variables. In partners, Type D personality was independently associatedwith increased symptoms of anxiety (OR: 8.77; 95% CI: 3.19-24.14) and depression (OR: 4.40; 95% CI: 1.76-11.01).
Aquarius AE. Role of disease status and Type D personality in outcomes in patients with peripheral arterial disease.	150	Patients with peripheral arterial disease were assessed with the Type D Scale-14, World Health Organization Quality of Life Assessment Instrument-100, and Perceived Stress Scale-10 Item assessed type D personality, QOL, and perceived stress	Type D patients reported significantly poorer quality of life than non-type D patients across peripheral arterial disease and healthy subgroups (p < 0.0001). After controlling for disease status (presence or absence of peripheral arterial disease), type D personality remained associated with increased risk for impaired quality of life (odds ratio [OR] 7.35, 95% confidence interval [CI] 3.39 to 15.96, p < 0.0001) and perceived stress (OR 6.45, 95% CI 3.42 to 12.18, p < 0.0001).
Denollet J. Personality, disease severity, and the risk of long-term cardiac events in patients with a decreased ejection fraction after myocardial infarction.	87	Patients with myocardial infarction with a decreased left ventricular ejection fraction (LVEF).	Patients with Type D personality were more likely to experience an event over time compared with non-type D patients (P=0.00005). Cox proportional hazards analysis yielded LVEF of < or =30% (relative risk, 3.0; 95% confidence interval, 1.2 to 7.7; P=.02) and type D (relative risk, 4.7; 95% confidence interval, 1.9 to 11.8; P=0.001) as independent predictors.
Denollet J. Unfavorable outcome of heart transplantation in recipients with type D personality.	51	Patients with transplanted heart were identified to have or not to have Type D personality by using the DS14 scale.	Type D recipients had a 10-fold higher mortality rate after hospital discharge (5 of 15, or 33%) as compared with non-Type D recipients (1 of 34, or 3%) (p = 0.013, adjusting for age and gender). Among surviving recipients, the rate of Grade "/> or =3A rejection for both groups was 40% vs 27%, respectively (p = 0.45). The risk of unfavorable outcomes (death, Grade "/> or =3A rejection, or number rejection-free days < or =14) was greater in Type D recipients (12 of 15, or 80%) than in

non-Type Ds (13 of 34, or 38%), adjusting for other risk factors (odds ratio: 6.75; 95% confidence interval: 1.47 to 30.97) (p = 0.014).

Table 3. Some important studies about negative affectivity and socal inhibition in cardiology

11. Education

Previous research showed that educational level is an important health determinant, with gender-related differences and ethnic and cultural variations. Low educated men and women, in particular with required schooling only, have usually low income and thus lower socio-economic status may be expected. The lower education level of older persons leads to greater burden for medical services and lower awareness of how to lead a healthy lifestyle, and lower adherence to medication and utilisation of preventive measures. In general, women take part more often in screening programs, are more interested in health prevention and visit their general practitioners more often. Their activity may also relate to a higher rate of diagnosis of depression and anxiety disorders. Besides biological factors including oestradiol, psychosocial factors, culture and education may be responsible for the prevalence of these mental disorders among women [66]. Less education was showed an important risk factor for late-life depression [67]. In survey in South America women's higher education was associated with lower risk for diabetes and hypertension and lower BMI in all areas but more strongly in urban areas. There was no association or even an adverse association between education and these risk factors among men in less urban areas [68]. Controversially, men with low level of education were related to higher BMI, prevalence of diabetes and smoking. Less-educated women had higher blood pressure and BMI and low education in both sexes was associated with twofold increased incidence of stroke and CHD [69]. In an Austrian study both men and women with lower educational levels were associated with unhealthy behaviours, overweight and higher cardiovascular risk. There was in inverse relationship in both men and women between overweight and obesity and educational level. The odds of daily smoking, eating a diet rich in meat and doing no regular vigorous exercise decreased with increasing educational level. Among women, the odds of suffering from diabetes or from hypertension decreased gradually with increasing educational level. There was no clear association between educational level and the risk of diabetes or hypertension in men. Depression among women with only required schooling was frequent, but showed no relationship with education in men [66]. Low education and income are important determinants of all-cause mortality and cardiovascular mortality [70] among patients with myocardial infarction. Low income and education are related to a higher risk profile and poorer treatment [71]. In accordance, in our study, a higher level of education was associated with a longer survival time after CABG. Those patients who had an academic degree had a mean survival time of 8.01 years, patients with 9 to 12 years of education had a mean survival time of 7.73 years and the group with 8 years or less of education had a mean survival time of 7.03 years. There were significant differences among patients with 8 years or less of education and patients with 8 to 12 years of education and patients with an academic degree in the survival analysis. Patients with less education had a worse life expectancy. There was no significant difference between patients with 9 to 12 years of education and those with an academic degree [13]. Patients with a high level of education are likely to have a higher income and therefore can afford the more expensive "healthy" diet and sport activities [70]. In a recent study, however, the risk for major cardiac event after primary percutaneous coronary intervention depended only on employment status and income, but not education level [72]. More prospective studies are needed to establish the relationship.

12. Interventions

The American Heart Association has recommended routine screening by self- reporting measures to rapid identification of likely depressed CAD patients. The Patient Health Questionnaire is one such depression assessing measurement, focuses on two requisite symptoms for a depression or major depressive episode diagnosis, i.e., (1) little interest or pleasure in doing things, (2) feeling down, depressed, or hopeless. Patients with positive screening results should be evaluated by a professional qualified in the diagnosis and management of depression [5].

12.1. Antidepressants

There are currently several empirically validated treatments for depression. A national survey of cardiovascular physicians reported nearly 50% of respondents treat the symptoms of depression once identified in patients with CAD [73]. The Selective serotonin re-uptake inhibitors (SSRI) are currently considered the safest to use with CAD patients, in contrast to the tricyclics, which may have pro-arrhythmic and cardio-toxic effects. The SSRI have been hypothesized as safe among cardiac patients due to the serotonin transporter affinity and attenuation of platelet functioning. The SADHART trial compared the effects of sertraline and placebo for 24 weeks in major depressive patients with unstable angina or recent MI. The SSRI treatment did not adversely affect cardiac function and was considered to be safe for most patients [74]. However, in the ENRICHD trial, improvements in depression were rather modest. Patients with at least 1 prior episode of depression or more severe depression showed consistent improvement in depression relative to control, suggesting that treatment with SSRIs is a good option for this subset of depressed CAD patients. The ENRICHD trial also found that antidepressant treatment improved prognosis for myocardial infarction patients, they were at decreased risk for death and reinfarction compared with those who did not take antidepressants [75]. In a systematic review [76] only 2 studies had follow-up periods that were long enough to assess cardiac outcomes [76, 77]. None of them found evidence of an effect of depression treatment. Two studies reported that selective serotonin reuptake inhibitors did not affect cardiac function [74, 79]. Possible side effects of SSRIs for CABG surgery patients include increased bleeding, but have not been consistently supported [80]. One study suggested an increased long-term mortality and rehospitalization after CABG surgery attributable to SSRIs [81]. Another study indicated greater renal morbidity and ventilation times, but not greater mortality or bleeding risk [82]. In two recent systematic reviews of randomized, controlled trials in CAD patients both established SSRI vs. placebo there was no difference i mortality and differential findings were reported on hospital readmissions. One found reduced odds [83], whereas another review did not when applying stringent criteria for properly randomized studies [84]. There is no trial about the role of anxiolytic drugs before or after CABG with or without concomitant depressive symptoms.

12.2. Psychosocial Interventions

Psychosocial interventions (psychotherapy, support, stress reduction) have been used as treatments for depression in CAD patients. The aim of these interventions is to reduce psychological distress, which in theory would ultimately improve clinical outcomes. Patients with depression often do not participate or complete cardiac rehabilitation programs after CABG and thus may form a barrier to improvements in cardiac functioning [85]. From another aspect, isolated patients may be difficult to enroll in interventions because they do feel that they have a problem. Without the experience of need, motivation to change may be low [86]. Numerous behavioural and psychological randomized controlled trial (RCT) interventions have been reported and cognitive behavioural therapy or collaborative care constitutes Class IIa evidence (i.e., it is reasonable to administer treatment, additional studies with focused objectives are needed) [85]. In one of RCT studies on brief, tailored cognitive behavioural therapy targeting preoperative depression and anxiety researchers found that intervention improved depressive and anxiety symptoms, as well as quality of life. Moreover, it reduced in-hospital length of stay [87]. In a Canadian study eight weeks prior to CABG, the treatment group received exercise training twice per week, education and reinforcement, and monthly nurse-initiated telephone calls. After surgery, participation in a cardiac rehabilitation program was offered to all patients. The intervention was not associated with differences in pre-surgery anxiety versus usual care, however length of stay differed significantly between groups. Patients who received the preoperative intervention spent 1 less day in the hospital overall and less time in the intensive care. During the waiting period, patients in the intervention group had a better quality of life than controls. Improved quality of life continued up to 6 months after surgery. Mortality rates did not differ [88]. In a prospective randomized controlled trial the effects of a home-based intervention program on anxiety and depression 6 months after CABG were assessed. Anxiety and depression symptoms were measured before surgery, 6 weeks after surgery, and 6 months after surgery. On 6-week and 6-month follow-ups, significant improvements in anxiety and depression symptoms were found in both groups. There was no significant difference between patients receiving interventions and not [89]. Freedland et al. compared cognitive behaviour or supportive stress management vs usual care and found significant three month depression remission rates in the treatment arms. Cognitive behaviour therapy had greater and more durable effects than supportive stress management on depression and several secondary psychological outcomes [90]. The limitation of psychosocial RCTs among CABG populations is that those patients experiencing significant postoperative morbidity are likely to be excluded from trial inclusion. Therefore, less is known about long term outcomes for patients who experience stroke, deep sternal wound infection, sternal dehiscence, renal failure requiring dialysis and extended length of time on mechanical ventilation, or intensive care during their hospital stay. These moribund patients are at higher risks for developing or exacerbating psychological distress. Moreover, treatment of affective disorders is important in any context, there is not sufficient evidence whether interventions among cardiac patients can promote and maintain health related behaviour change [25]. Exercise is commonly recommended to promote both primary and secondary CAD prevention, but evidence suggests that exercise may also modify psychosocial risk factors, including depression. Cross sectional studies of both patients and healthy cohorts have consistently demonstrated lower depression rates among those who are most active [55]. A randomized controlled comparison between antidepressant medication versus exercise was performed in depressed patients. After 16 weeks, there was a significant reduction in depression in all groups, confirming the same effect of exercise and sertraline hydrochloride in reducing depressive symptoms. However, a lower rate of relapse was observed in the exercise group after six months [91].

13. Conclusion and future directions

Coronary artery bypass graft surgery (CABG) is a confirmed procedure to relive angina pectoris and reduce the risk from life-threatening ischaemic heart disease, besides reducing the likelihood of future heart attacks and prolonging life-expectancy. Another goal is to improve health-related quality of life and psychological well-being. After successful surgery the majority of patients can have an improved everyday life, with increased performance in physical, social and sexual functioning and decreased levels of depression, anxiety, fatigue and sleep. In some cases quality of life for patients can be disappointing, and attention has increasingly been paid to psychological difficulties following CABG surgery [92]. Psychological problems such as depression and anxiety are widely reported soon after CABG surgery and remain evident for around one-fifth of patients one year after surgery. Poor psychological adjustment following surgery can increase the likelihood of new coronary events, further hospitalisations and even death. According to a recent study 30% of patients have reduced health related quality of life without being clinically anxious or depressed they present with fear of activity, fear of excitement, give up enjoyed hobbies / activities. Evidence suggests that self-perceived health related quality of life, depressive symptoms and anxiety together influence the short and long term recovery following coronary bypass surgery [93]. There is also a higher risk for morbidity and mortality among the lonely and the socially isolated, they are likely to have prolonged postoperative recovery and hospital stay. Lower education and poor social background are associated with higher mortality rates related to CHD and prolonged hospital stay after CABG [93, 94]. Further research on the interaction between these disorders and social factors may improve our understandings and uncover promising ways for intervention. Most studies to date focus on depression, the role of other factors alone or investigated together warrants further research.

In conclusion, compared with community samples the prevalence of depression and anxiety disorders are significantly higher and they confer greater morbidity risks, though the behavioural and biological mechanisms are poorly understood. Researchers and clinicians hope psychosocial intervention might decrease or cease the deleterious impact of depression and anxiety on morbidity and mortality.

Author details

Zsuzsanna Cserép[1], Andrea Székely[1,2] and Bela Merkely[3]

*Address all correspondence to: szekelya@kardio.hu

1 Department of Anesthesiology and Intensive Care, Semmelweis University, Budapest, Hungary and Uzsoki Street Hospital of the Budapest Municipality, Budapest, Hungary

2 Intensive Care, Gottsegen György Hungarian Institute of Cardiology, Budapest, Hungary

3 Department of Cardiology, Semmelweis University, Budapest, Hungary

References

[1] Krannich JH, Weyers P, Lueger S, Herzog M, Bohrer T, Elert O. Presence of depression and anxiety before and after coronary artery bypass graft surgery and their relationship to age. BMC Psychiatry. 2007;7:47.

[2] Rozanski A, Blumenthal JA, Davidson KW, Saab PG, Kubzansky L. The epidemiology, pathophysiology, and management of psychosocial risk factors in cardiac practice: the emerging field of behavioral cardiology. J Am Coll Cardiol. 2005;45:637-51.

[3] Blumenthal JA, Lett HS, Babyak MA, White W, Smith PK, Mark DB, et al; NORG Investigators. Depression as a risk factor for mortality after coronary artery bypass surgery. Lancet, 2003;362:604-9.

[4] Connerney I, Shapiro PA, McLaughlin JS, Bagiella E, Sloan RP. Relation between depression after coronary artery bypass surgery and 12-month outcome: a prospective study. Lancet. 2001;358:1766-71.

[5] Lichtman JH, Bigger JT Jr, Blumenthal JA, Frasure-Smith N, Kaufmann PG, Lespérance F, et al; American Heart Association Prevention Committee of the Council on Cardiovascular Nursing; American Heart Association Council on Clinical Cardiology; American Heart Association Council on Epidemiology and Prevention; American Heart Association Interdisciplinary Council on Quality of Care and Outcomes Research; American Psychiatric Association. Depression and coronary heart disease: recommendations for screening, referral, and treatment: a science advisory from the American Heart Association Prevention Committee of the Council on Cardiovascular Nursing, Council on Clinical Cardiology, Council on Epidemiology and Prevention, and Interdisciplinary Council on Quality of Care and Outcomes Research: endorsed by the American Psychiatric Association. Circulation. 2008;118:1768-75.

[6] Majed B, Arveiler D, Bingham A, Ferrieres J, Ruidavets JB, Montaye M, et al; PRIME Study Group. Depressive symptoms, a time-dependent risk factor for coronary heart disease and stroke in middle-aged men: the PRIME Study. Strokc. 2012;43:1761-7.

[7] Barefoot JC, Helms MJ, Mark DB, Blumenthal JA, Califf RM, Haney TL, et al. Depression and long-term mortality risk in patients with coronary artery disease. Am J Cardiol. 1996;78:613–7.

[8] Frasure-Smith N, Lesperance F, Juneau M, Talajic M, Bourassa MG. Gender, depression, and one-year prognosis after myocardial infarction. Psychosom Med. 1999;61:26–37.

[9] Lesperance F, Frasure-Smith N, Talajic M, Bourassa MG. Five-year risk of cardiac mortality in relation to initial severity and one-year changes in depression symptoms after myocardial infarction. Circulation. 2002;105:1049 –53.

[10] Brown JM, Stewart JC, Stump TE, Callahan CM. Risk of coronary heart disease events over 15 years among older adults with depressive symptoms. Am J Geriatr Psychiatry. 2011;19:721-9.

[11] Mahoney JJ, Voelkel EA, Bannister JA, Gopaldas RR, Dao TK. Psychiatric Factors Which Impact Coronary Heart Disease and Influence Outcomes Post-Coronary Artery Bypass Grafting Surgery. Rijeka: In Tech; 2012. http://www.intechopen.com/ books/howtoreference/front-lines-of-thoracic-surgery/psychiatric-factors-which-impact-coronary-heart-disease-chd-and-influence-outcomes-post-coronary-art   (accessed 11 October 2012).

[12] Tully PJ, Baker RA, Turnbull D, Winefield H. The role of depression and anxiety symptoms in hospital readmissions after cardiac surgery. J Behav Med. 2008;31:281-90.

[13] Cserep Z, Losoncz E, Balog P, Szili-Török T, Husz A, Juhász B, et al. The impact of preoperative anxiety and education level on long-term mortality after cardiac surgery. J Cardiothorac Surg. 2012;7(1):86.

[14] Fava M, Abraham M, Pava J, Shuster J, Rosenbaum J. Cardiovascular risk factors in depression: the role of anxiety and anger. Psychosomatics. 1996;37:31-37.

[15] Esler M, Turbott J, Schwarz R, Leonard P, Bobik A, Skews H, et al. The peripheral kinetics of norepinephrine in depressive illness. Arch Gen Psychiatry. 1982;39:285-300.

[16] Watkins LL, Grossman P, Krishnan R, Sherwood A. Anxiety and vagal control of heart risk. Psychosom Med. 1998;60:498-502.

[17] Kawachi I, Sparrow D, Vokonas PS, Weiss ST. Decreased heart rate variability in men with phobic anxiety (data from the Normative Aging Study). Am J Cardiol. 1995;75:882-885.

[18] van Boven AJ, Jukema JW, Haaksma J, Zwinderman AH, Crijns HJ, Lie KI. Depressed heart rate variability is associated with events in patients with stable coronary artery disease and preserved left ventricular function. REGRESS Study Group. Am Heart J. 1998;135:571-576.

[19] Krantz D, Helmers K, Bairey CN, Nebel L, Hedges S, Rozanski A. Cardiovascular reactivity and mental stress-induced myocardial ischemia in patients with coronary artery disease. Psychosom Med. 1991;53:1-12.

[20] Carney RM, Freedland KE, Rich MW, Jaffe AS. Depression as a risk factor for cardiac events in established coronary heart disease: a review of possible mechanisms. Ann Behav Med. 1995;17:142-149.

[21] Roest AM, Martens EJ, Denollet J, de Jonge P. Prognostic association of anxiety post myocardial infarction with mortality and new cardiac events: a meta-analysis. Psychosom Med. 2010;72:563-9.

[22] Everson-Rose SA, Lewis TT. Psychosocial factors and cardiovascular diseases. Annu Rev Public Health. 2005;26:469-500.

[23] Frasure-Smith N, Lesperance F. Depression and other psychological risks following myocardial infarction. Arch. Gen. Psychiatry 2003; 60:627–36.

[24] Koivula M, Tarkka MT, Tarkka M, Laippala P, Paunonen-Ilmonen M. Fear and anxiety in patients at different time-points in the coronary artery bypass process. Int J Nurs Stud. 2002;39:811-22.

[25] Tully PJ, Baker RA. Depression, anxiety, and cardiac morbidity outcomes after coronary artery bypass surgery: a contemporary and practical review. J Geriatr Cardiol. 2012;9:197-208.

[26] Rosenbloom JI, Wellenius GA, Mukamal KJ, Mittleman MA. Self-reported anxiety and the risk of clinical events and atherosclerotic progression among patients with Coronary Artery Bypass Grafts (CABG). Am Heart J. 2009;158:867-73.

[27] Székely A, Balog P, Benkö E, Breuer T, Székely J, Kertai MD, et al. Anxiety predicts mortality and morbidity after coronary artery and valve surgery--a 4-year follow-up study. Psychosom Med. 2007;69(7):625-31.

[28] Kawachi I, Sparrow D, Vokonas PS, Weiss ST. Symptoms of anxiety and risk of coronary heart disease. The Normative Aging Study. Circulation. 1994; 90:2225-9.

[29] Dao TK, Voelkel E, Presley S, Doss B, Huddleston C, Gopaldas R. Gender as a moderator between having an anxiety disorder diagnosis and coronary artery bypass grafting surgery (CABG) outcomes in rural patients. J Rural Health. 2012;28:260-7.

[30] Oxlad M, Stubberfield J, Stuklis R, Edwards J, Wade TD. Psychological risk factors for cardiac-related hospital readmission within 6 months of coronary artery bypass graft surgery. J Psychosom Res. 2006;61:775-81.

[31] Kopp MS, Skrabski Á, Réthelyi J, Kawachi I, Adler N. Self Rated Health, Subjective Social Status and Middle Aged Mortality in a Changing Society. Behav Med. 2004;30:65-70.

[32] Jylhä M, Volpato S, Guralnik JM. Self-rated health showed a graded association with frequently used biomarkers in a large population sample. J Clin Epidemiol. 2006;59:465-71.

[33] Jylhä M. What is self-rated health and why does it predict mortality? Towards a unified conceptual model. Soc Sci Med. 2009;69:307-16.

[34] Arnadottir SA, Gunnarsdottir ED, Stenlund H, Lundin-Olsson L. Determinants of self-rated health in old age: a population-based, cross-sectional study using the International Classification of Functioning. BMC Public Health. 2011;11:670.

[35] Schroeder S, Baumbach A, Herdeg C, Oberhoff M, Buchholz O, Kuettner A, et al. Self-rated health and clinical status after PTCA: results of a 4-year follow-up in 500 patients. Eur J Intern Med. 2001;12:101-106.

[36] Norekvål TM, Fridlund B, Rokne B, Segadal L, Wentzel-Larsen T, Nordrehaug JE. Patient-reported outcomes as predictors of 10-year survival in women after acute myocardial infarction. Health Qual Life Outcomes. 2010;8:140.

[37] Oxlad M, Wade TD. Longitudinal risk factors for adverse psychological functioning six months after coronary artery bypass graft surgery. J Health Psychol. 2008;13:79-92.

[38] Steptoe A, Wardle J, Marmot M. Positive affect and health-related neuroendocrine, cardiovascular, and inflammatory processes. Proc Natl Acad Sci USA. 2005;102:6508-12.

[39] Steptoe A, Dockray S, Wardle J. Positive affect and psychobiological processes relevant to health. J Pers. 2009;77:1747-76.

[40] Kubzansky LD, Thurston RC. Emotional vitality and incident coronary heart disease: benefits of healthy psychological functioning. Arch Gen Psychiatry. 2007;64:1393-401.

[41] Scheier MF, Matthews KA, Owens JF, Schulz R, Bridges MW, Magovern GJ, et al. Optimism and rehospitalization after coronary artery bypass graft surgery. Arch Intern Med. 1999;159:829-35.

[42] Tindle H, Belnap BH, Houck PR, Mazumdar S, Scheier MF, Matthews KA, et al. Optimism, response to treatment of depression, and rehospitalization after coronary artery bypass graft surgery. Psychosom Med. 2012;74:200-7.

[43] Devins GM. Using the illness intrusiveness ratings scale to understand health-related quality of life in chronic disease. J Psychosom Res. 2010;68:591-602.

[44] Cserép Z, Balog P, Székely J, Treszl A, Kopp MS, Thayer JF, et al. Psychosocial factors and major adverse cardiac and cerebrovascular events after cardiac surgery. Interact Cardiovasc Thorac Surg. 2010;11:567-72.

[45] Czajkowski SM. Health-related quality of life outcomes in clinical research: NHLBI policy and perspectives. Ann Thorac Surg. 1998;66:1486-7.

[46] Koch CG, Li L, Lauer M, Sabik J, Starr NJ, Blackstone EH. Effect of functional health-related quality of life on long-term survival after cardiac surgery. Circulation. 2007;115:692-9.

[47] Rumsfeld JS, MaWhinney S, McCarthy M Jr, Shroyer AL, VillaNueva CB, O'Brien M, et al. Health-related quality of life as a predictor of mortality following coronary artery bypass graft surgery. Participants of the Department of Veterans Affairs Cooperative Study Group on Processes, Structures, and Outcomes of Care in Cardiac Surgery. JAMA. 1999;281:1298-303.

[48] Vaccarino V. Women and outcomes of coronary artery bypass surgery: do we have an answer? Am Heart J. 2003;146:935-7.

[49] Koch CG, Nussmeier NA. Gender and cardiac surgery. Anesthesiol Clin North America. 2003;21:675-89.

[50] Lindquist R, Dupuis G, Terrin ML, Hoogwerf B, Czajkowski S, Herd JA, et al; POST CABG Biobehavioral Study Investigators. Comparison of health-related quality-of-life outcomes of men and women after coronary artery bypass surgery through 1 year: findings from the POST CABG Biobehavioral Study. Am Heart J. 2003;146:1038-44.

[51] Phillips Bute B, Mathew J, Blumenthal JA, Welsh-Bohmer K, White WD, Mark D, et al. Female gender is associated with impaired quality of life 1 year after coronary artery bypass surgery. Psychosom Med. 2003;65:944-51.

[52] Herlitz J, Wiklund I, Caidahl K, Hartford M, Haglid M, Karlsson BW, et al. The feeling of loneliness prior to coronary artery bypass grafting might be a predictor of short-and long-term postoperative mortality. Eur J Vasc Endovasc Surg. 1998;16:120-5.

[53] Balog P, Janszky I, Leineweber C, Blom M, Wamala SP, Orth-Gomér K. Depressive symptoms in relation to marital and work stress in women with and without coronary heart disease. The Stockholm Female Coronary Risk Study. Journal of Psychosomatic Research. 2003;54:113-9.

[54] Balog P, Mészáros E. Házastársi stressz, depressziós tünetek és a cardiovascularis vulnerabilitás - nőknél. LAM. 2005;8:685-92.

[55] Rozanski A, Blumenthal JA, Kaplan J. Impact of psychological factors on the pathogenesis of cardiovascular disease and implications for therapy. Circulation. 1999;99:2192–217.

[56] Kopp MS, Skrabski A, Székely A, Stauder A, Williams R. Chronic stress and social changes: socioeconomic determination of chronic stress. Ann N Y Acad Sci. 2007;1113:325-38.

[57] Orth-Gomer K, Wamala SP, Horsten M, Schenck-Gustafsson K, Schneiderman N, Mittleman MA. Marital stress worsens prognosis in women with coronary heart disease: the Stockholm Female Coronary Risk Study. JAMA 2000;284:3008 –14.

[58] Gallo LC, Troxel WM, Kuller LH, Sutton-Tyrrell K, Edmundowicz D, Matthews KA. Marital status, marital quality, and atherosclerotic burden in postmenopausal women. Psychosom Med 2003;65:952– 62.

[59] Denollet J. DS14: standard assessment of negative affectivity, social inhibition, and Type D personality. Psychosom Med. 2005;67:89-97.

[60] Denollet J, Sys SU, Stroobant N, Rombouts H, Gillebert TC, Brutsaert DL. Personality as independent predictor of long-term mortality in patients with coronary heart disease. Lancet. 1996;347:417–21.

[61] Pedersen SS, Lemos PA, van Vooren PR, Liu TK, Daemen J, Erdman RA, et al. Type D personality predicts death or myocardial infarction after bare metal stent or sirolimus-eluting stent implantation: a Rapamycin-Eluting Stent Evaluated At Rotterdam Cardiology Hospital (RESEARCH) registry sub-study. J Am Coll Cardiol. 2004;44:997– 1001.

[62] Pedersen SS, van Domburg RT, Theuns DA, Jordaens L, Erdman RA. Type D personality is associated with increased anxiety and depressive symptoms in patients with an implantable cardioverter defibrillator and their partners. Psychosom Med. 2004;66:714– 9.

[63] Aquarius AE, Denollet J, Hamming JF, De Vries J. Role of disease status and Type D personality in outcomes in patients with peripheral arterial disease. Am J Cardiol. 2005;96:996–1001.

[64] Denollet J, Brutsaert DL. Personality, disease severity, and the risk of long-term cardiac events in patients with a decreased ejection fraction after myocardial infarction. Circulation. 1998;97:167-73.

[65] Denollet J, Holmes RV, Vrints CJ, Conraads VM. Unfavorable outcome of heart transplantation in recipients with type D personality. J Heart Lung Transplant. 2007;26:152-8.

[66] Kautzky-Willer A, Dorner T, Jensby A, Rieder A. Women show a closer association between educational level and hypertension or diabetes mellitus than males: a secondary analysis from the Austrian HIS. BMC Public Health. 2012;12:392.

[67] Chang-Quan H, Zheng-Rong W, Yong-Hong L, Yi-Zhou X, Qing-Xiu L. Review Education and risk for late life depression: a meta-analysis of published literature. Int J Psychiatry Med. 2010; 40:109-24.

[68] Fleischer NL, Diez Roux AV, Alazraqui M, Spinelli H, De Maio F. Socioeconomic gradients in chronic disease risk factors in middle-income countries: evidence of effect modification by urbanicity in Argentina. Am J Public Health. 2011;101:294-301.

[69] Veronesi G, Ferrario MM, Chambless LE, Sega R, Mancia G, Corrao G, et al. Gender differences in the association between education and the incidence of cardiovascular events in Northern Italy. Eur J Public Health. 2011;21:762-7.

[70] Kopp M, Skrabski A, Szántó Z, Siegrist J. Psychosocial determinants of premature cardiovascular mortality differences within Hungary. J Epidemiol Community Health. 2006;60:782 88.

[71] Gerber Y, Goldbourt U, Drory Y, Israel Study Group on First Acute Myocardial Infarction: Interaction between income and education in predicting long-term survival after acute myocardial infarction. Eur J Cardiovasc Prev Rehabil. 2008;15:526–32.

[72] Jakobsen L, Niemann T, Thorsgaard N, Thuesen L, Lassen JF, Jensen LO, et al. Dimensions of Socioeconomic Status and Clinical Outcome After Primary Percutaneous Coronary Intervention. Circ Cardiovasc Interv. 2012 Oct http://circinterventions.ahajournals.org/content/early/2012/10/02/CIRCINTERVENTIONS. 112.968271.long (accessed 11 October 2012.)

[73] Feinstein RE, Blumenfield M, Orlowski B, Frishman WH, Ovanessian S. A national survey of cardiovascular physicians' beliefs and clinical care practices when diagnosing and treating depression in patients with cardiovascular disease. Cardiol Rev. 2006;14(4):164-9.

[74] Glassman AH, O'Connor CM, Califf RM, Swedberg K, Schwartz P, Bigger JT, et al, SADHEART Group. Sertraline treatment of major depression in patients with acute MI or unstable angina. JAMA. 2002;288:701–9.

[75] Writing committee for the ENRICHD investigators. Effects of treating depression and low social support on clinical events after myocardial infarction: The enhancing recovery in coronary heart disease patients (ENRICHD) randomized trial. JAMA. 2003;289:3106–16.

[76] Thombs BD, de Jonge P, Coyne JC, Whooley MA, Frasure-Smith N, Mitchell AJ, et al. Depression screening and patient outcomes in cardiovascular care: a systematic review. JAMA. 2008;300:2161-71.

[77] Berkman LF, Blumenthal J, Burg M, Carney RM, Catellier D, Cowan MJ, et al; Enhancing Recovery in Coronary Heart Disease Patients Investigators (ENRICHD). Effects of treating depression and low perceived social support on clinical events after myocardial infarction: the Enhancing Recovery in Coronary Heart Disease patients (ENRICHD) randomized trial. JAMA. 2003;289:3106-3116.

[78] van Melle JP, de Jonge P, Honig A, Schene AH, Kuyper AM, Crijns HJ, et al; MIND-IT investigators. Effects of antidepressant treatment following myocardial infarction. Br J Psychiatry. 2007;190:460-66.

[79] Strik JJ, Honig A, Lousberg R, Lousberg AH, Cheriex EC, Tuynman-Qua HG, et al. Efficacy and safety of fluoxetine in the treatment of patients with major depression after first myocardial infarction: findings from a double-blind, placebo-controlled trial. Psychosom Med. 2000;62:783-89.

[80] Lett HS, Blumenthal JA, Babyak MA, Sherwood A, Strauman T, Robins C, et al. Depression as a risk factor for coronary artery disease: evidence, mechanisms, and treatment. Psychosom Med. 2004;66:305-15.

[81] Xiong GL, Jiang W, Clare R, Shaw LK, Smith PK, Mahaffey KW, et al. Prognosis of patients taking selective serotonin reuptake inhibitors before coronary artery bypass grafting. Am J Cardiol. 2006;98:42-7.

[82] Tully PJ, Cardinal T, Bennetts JS, Baker RA. Selective serotonin reuptake inhibitors, venlafaxine and duloxetine are associated with in hospital morbidity but not bleeding or late mortality after coronary artery bypass graft surgery. Heart Lung Circ. 2012; 21:206-14.

[83] Baumeister H, Hutter N, Bengel J. Review Psychological and pharmacological interventions for depression in patients with coronary artery disease. Cochrane Database Syst Rev. 2011; (9):CD008012.

[84] Pizzi C, Rutjes AW, Costa GM, Fontana F, Mezzetti A, Manzoli L. Meta-analysis of selective serotonin reuptake inhibitors in patients with depression and coronary heart disease. Am J Cardiol. 2011; 107:972-9.

[85] Hillis LD, Smith PK, Anderson JL, Bittl JA, Bridges CR, Byrne JG, et al. 2011 ACCF/AHA Guideline for Coronary Artery Bypass Graft Surgery: Executive Summary A Report of the American College of Cardiology Foundation/American Heart Association Task Force on Practice Guidelines Developed in Collaboration With the American Association for Thoracic Surgery, Society of Cardiovascular Anesthesiologists, and Society of Thoracic Surgeons. J Am Coll Cardiol. 2011;58:2584-614.

[86] Brummett BH, Barefoot JC, Siegler IC, Clapp-Channing NE, Lytle BL, Bosworth HB, et al. Characteristics of socially isolated patients with coronary artery disease who are at elevated risk for mortality. Psychosom Med. 2001;63:267-72.

[87] Dao TK, Youssef NA, Armsworth M, Wear E, Papathopoulos KN, Gopaldas R. Randomized controlled trial of brief cognitive behavioral intervention for depression and anxiety symptoms preoperatively in patients undergoing coronary artery bypass graft surgery. J Thorac Cardiovasc Surg. 2011;142:e109-15.

[88] Arthur HM, Daniels C, McKelvie R, Hirsh J, Rush B. Effect of a preoperative intervention on preoperative and postoperative outcomes in low-risk patients awaiting

elective coronary artery bypass graft surgery. A randomized, controlled trial. Ann Intern Med. 2000;133:253-62.

[89] Lie I, Arnesen H, Sandvik L, Hamilton G, Bunch EH. Effects of a home-based intervention program on anxiety and depression 6 months after coronary artery bypass grafting: a randomized controlled trial. J Psychosom Res. 2007;62:411-8.

[90] Freedland KE, Skala JA, Carney RM, Rubin EH, Lustman PJ, Dávila-Román VG, et al. Treatment of depression after coronary artery bypass surgery: a randomized controlled trial. Arch Gen Psychiatry. 2009;66:387-96.

[91] Babyak M, Blumenthal JA, Herman S, Khatri P, Doraiswamy M, Moore K, et al. Exercise treatment for major depression: maintenance of therapeutic benefit at 10 months. Psychosom Med. 2000;62:633– 8.

[92] McKenzie LH, Simpson J, Stewart M. A systematic review of pre-operative predictors of post-operative depression and anxiety in individuals who have undergone coronary artery bypass graft surgery. Psychol Health Med. 2010;15:74-93.

[93] Cserép Z, Losoncz E, Malik A, Székely A, Balog P, Kopp M. Psychosocial factors determining life expectancy of patients undergoing open heart surgery. Orv Hetil. 2008;149:1549-54.

[94] Johnston G, Goss JR, Malmgren JA, Spertus JA. Health Status and Social Risk Correlates of Extended Length of Stay Following CABG Surgery. Ann Thorac Surg. 2004;77:557-62.

Chapter 10

Current Challenges in the Treatment of Deep Sternal Wound Infection Following Cardiac Surgery

Martin Šimek, Martin Molitor, Martin Kaláb,
Patrick Tobbia and Vladimír Lonský

Additional information is available at the end of the chapter

1. Introduction

Median sternotomy due to its technical simplicity and excellent exposure of the heart, great vessels and pulmonary hila is the most common incision performed in cardiothoracic surgery worldwide [1]. Originally described by Julian more than 100 years ago and re-induced by Milton in 1957, median sternotomy replaced gradually thoracotomy or bilateral transverse sternothoracotomy (clamshell incision) for routine access to the heart [2,3]. Even though median sternotomy is still considered to be the gold standard, efforts remain ongoing to use less invasive methods such as partial sternotomy or small thoracotomy to influence the risk of wound healing complications, patient's satisfaction and better quality of life [4].

2. Incidence and risk factors of Deep Sternal Wound Infection (DSWI)

Infection involving the sternal bones and/or retrosternal space is a serious complication of median sternotomy. Although, DSWI can be described from many perspectives, the definition according to the Center for Disease Control and Prevention (CDC), is used for distinguishing DSWI from others types of sternal wound infections (SWIs), and is respected by most authors (Table 1) [5]. Looking through the incidence of DSWI ranging between 0.3 to 3.2%, no considerable changes have been observed in the incidence of DSWI over the last 30 years [6-22]. It could be perceived that the numerous advances in cardiac surgery, post-operative care and employment of preventive measurements may have played a role in reducing the incidence of DSWI in the last 10 years. Today surgically treated patients' cohorts are different than patients operated on 20 years ago in terms of advanced age, co-morbidities, and surgical complexity. In other words, the relatively steady status of DSWI incidence over the last three decades might be considered a satisfactory result [23]. Recently Matros et al showed from a large single institution experience with 21,000 sternotomies a reduction in the incidence of DSWI from 1.57 to 0.88% in the last 15 years. They concluded that the rate of DSWI was significantly diminished particularly in the diabetic population, from 3.2% to 1.0%, related to tight glycemic control [19].

Diagnosis of DSWI requires at least one of the following criteria:
(1) anorganism is isolated from culture of mediastinal tissue or fluid
(2) evidence of mediastinitis is seen during operation or byhistopathological examination
(3) one of the following, fever("/>38° C), chest pain, or sternal instability, is present
and there is either purulent drainage from the mediastinum
or an organism isolated from blood culture or culture of drainage of the mediastinal area

Table 1. Center for Disease Control and Prevention (CDC) criteria of DSWI (modified from Mangan et al[5])

The identification of risk factors for the development of DSWI is crucial in the effort to reduce the risk of infection [6-22]. Although more than two dozen factors were obtained for uni-, and multivariable analyses, only obesity and diabetes mellitus were constantly proven in published studies [6-18,21,22]. Obesity is a strong risk factor for development of DSWI. Even though BMI does not correlate closely with body fat, there is a step-wise relationship between BMI and the risk of major surgical infection in cardiac surgery [7,15,24]. It is caused not only through technical obesity-related problems, but also through less effective penetration of antibiotics into the fat tissue [24]. Undoubtedly, diabetics are at a higher risk of developing DSWI, making the role of perioperative glycemic control crucial. Unsatisfactory preoperative glycemic control is considered to be an important risk factor for development of DSWI [25,26]. Internal mammary artery (IMA) harvesting, particularly in the pedicled fashion, has been found to have a higher incidence of DSWI in a CABG cohort compared with valvular procedures [7,8]. Furthermore, this risk becomes stronger when both IMA are used for revascularization or in the diabetic population, but this effect might be attenuated when both IMA are taken down in a skeletonized fashion, even in diabetics [10,27,28]. Chronic obstructive pulmonary disease (COPD) or smoking increases the risk of infectious complications, prolonged post-operative ventilation, and jeopardizes sternal stability from excessive coughing [6,12,15]. Data addressing the impact of early tracheostomy on DSWI incidence is conflicting [29-31]. Historically, a strong relationship between early tracheostomy and DSWI has not been confirmed; but tracheostomy is known to reduce the need for mechanical ventilation and thereby may limit risk of pulmonary infection and ICU stay [32]. Furthermore, re-exploration for bleeding has been analyzed as an independent risk factor for DSWI in several studies [11,12]. The components of this risk factor include the risk of iatrogenic bacteriological wound contamination within the inherent re-exposure, the deleterious effect of anemia and/or concomitant hemodynamic instability, and the amount of given allogenic blood transfusion units [10,33]. Other factors traditionally associated with an increased risk of DSWI are inconsistently seen in analyses of retrospective studies including advanced age, emergency surgery, hemodynamic instability, low ejection fraction, duration of surgery and CPB time, and renal failure [6-22]. Incidence and risk factors based on multivariable analysis from larger retrospective studies are summarized in Table 2.

Authors	Patients' enrollment	No. of patients	DSWI incidence	Independent risk factors
Loop FD et al [6]	1985-1987	6504	1.1%	Obesity, BIMA+diabetes, time of operation,
Milano CA et al [7]	1987-1995	6459	1.3%	Obesity, CHF, re-do surgery, CPB time
Braxton et al [8]	1992-1996	15406	1.25%	Obesity, low EF, COPD
Eklund et al [9]	1990-1999	10713	1.1%	Obesity, BMI
The Parisian Mediastinitis Study Group [10]	1996	1830	NA	Obesity, BIMA, hemodynamic instability, re-do surgery
Hollenbeak et al [11]	1996-1998	1519	2.7%	Obesity, renal inssuficieny, re-exploration
Filsouri et al [12]	1998-2005	5798	1.80%	Obesity, MI, diabetes, COPD, CPB time, re-exploration, prolonged ventilation
Tang et al [13]	1990-2003	30102	0.77%	Age, diabetes, stroke, CHF, BIMA +diabetes/CHF
Toumpoulis et al [14]	1992-2002	3760	1.1%	Diabetes,dialysis, hemodynamic instability, BIMA
Risnes et al [15]	1989-2000	18532	0.6%	Age, male gender, obesity, COPD, diabetes
Crabtree et al [16]	1996-2003	4004	2.2%	Obesity, diabetes,"/>2 transfusion units
Fowler et al [17]	2002-2003	331429	NA	Obesity, diabetes, MI, urgent surgery
Sjoegren et al [18]	1999-2004	4781	0.95%	Diabetes, obesity, low EF, renal failure
Matros et al [19]	1991-2006	21000	1.35%	Prolonged CPB time
De Feo et al [20]	1979-2009	22366	0.89%	NA
Upton et al [21]	1998-2003	5176	1.2%	Diabetes, urgent surgery, low EF
Sachithanandan et al [22]	2001-2005	4586	1.65%	Diabetes, smoking, age, prolonged ventilation

NA - not adrressed
BIMA - bilateral IMA harvesting
EF - ejection fraction
COPD - chronic obstructive pulmonary disease
CHF - congestive heart failure
MI - myocardial infaction

Table 2. Analyses of incidence and risk factors of DSWI

3. Microbiology of DSWI and routes of infection

Staphylococci, either S. aureus (SA) or coagulase-negative Staphylococcus (CONS) represent the most causative organism of DSWI, accounting for 60 to 80% of cases [34]. The proportion of individual strains of Staphylococcus and their methicillin-sensitivity varies between countries and institutions, reflecting their long-term hygienic and antibiotic policies [35]. Although surgical site infections are typically perceived to be an exogenous problem related to exposure to healthcare workers, the most causative pathogens are endogenous from patient's own skin or mucosal flora [36,37]. Nasal carriage of SA has been identified as a potential risk factor for DSWI [38], and genetically identical SA from nasal flora have been cultivated from sternotomy wounds [39]. Unlike SA which caused a more aggressive presentation, CONS infection accompanied with bacteremia as observed in 50-60% of cases [34, 40] had a rather indolent course, clinically manifested later, and was more prone to recurrence [41, 42]. DSWI is diagnosed in 40-70% of patients post-discharge, thus post-discharge surveillance of up to 90 days is recommended [43]. Gram negative strains contribute less commonly in the pathogenesis of DSWI and mostly translocate from other host site infections, such as pneumonia, urinary or abdominal infections [34]. Finally, no significant difference in mortality was observed between DSWI infections caused by CoNS, when compared to SA, or Gram-negative pathogens [34]. Mekontso-Dessap et al suggested that DSWI caused by methicillin-resistant SA (MRSA) may have worse actuarial survival than sensitive strains (MSSA) in terms of 1 month, 1-year, and 3- year survival (60.0%±12.6%, 52.5%±-3.4%, and 26.3%±19.7% versus 84.6% ±7.1%, 79.0%±8.6%, and 79.0%±-8.65, p=0.04), and a regression analysis revealed MRSA as an independent risk factor for overall mortality [44].

4. Outcomes and cost of DSWI

Unsurprisingly, DSWI negatively affected outcomes in cardiac surgery. Even with the adoption of modern treatment strategies, the reported in-hospital mortality for DSWI varies from 1.1 to 19% [6-9,11,16,45]. Although the mortality rate is similar to data reported from the 1980s, it appears that implementation of negative pressure wound therapy (NPWT) may improve long-term survival of patients [18,20,46]. Regardless of treatment strategy, in-hospital stay of DSWI patients is at least two weeks longer compared to patients with an uncomplicated post-operative course [6,10,11]. DSWI-related morbidity was repeatedly reported in relation to prolonged mechanical ventilation, renal impairment, atrial and ventricular arrhythmias, cerebrovascular accidents, need for hemodynamic support, and healing-related complications [20,47]. The cause of death in the early post-operative period is mostly multiple organ failure initiated by sepsis or specific DSWI-related complications such as serious bleeding [6-8,16,18, 20]. Predictors of a poor outcome in DSWI patients that have been reported include length of intensive care unit (ICU) stay, late indication for surgical revision, bacteremia, hemodynamic instability, and prolonged mechanical ventilation [47,48]. Loop et al presented the worse survival data of DSWI in patients operated on during the 1980s in comparison with a standard CABG population within a 3-year follow-up after surgery [6]. Survival analyses published in the last decade consistently confirm long-term complications of patients with mid-, and long term survival rates who were successfully treated for DSWI (Table 3) [8,11,12,14,15,18,22,46]. Specific reasons for worsening of long-term survival are not yet clear. Risnes et al reported significantly higher cardiac-related deaths in the post-DSWI group (34.6 vs. 21.4%, p<0.006) and poorer survival for males ten years after surgery [15]. In contrast with this data, Sjoegren et al and Bailot et al showed unimpaired long-term survival of DSWI patients in comparison with patients who had uncomplicated surgery once NPWT was used [18,46].

Authors	Patients´ enrollement	Survival analysis
Loop FD et al [6]	1985-1987	3-year survival of 62.5% compared to 69.0% survival for patients with positive cultures. Overall, the 3-year survival was 75%, which is significantly below previously reported 5-year and even 10-year survival for isolated coronary bypass patients
Braxton et al [8]	1992-1996	The adjusted survival rates at 30 days, 1 year, and 4 years were 93%, 78%, and 65% among patients with mediastinitis and 97%, 95%, and 89% without mediastinitis, respectively (p<0.001)
Hollenbeak et al [11]	1996-1998	DSWI patient had a 1-year survival of 78% vs. 99% for non-infected CABG patients, p=0.0001
Filsouri et al [12]	1998-2005	Survival rates at 1,3, and 5 years were 72.4%, 64.3% and 55.8% for patients with DSWI compared with 93.8%, 88% and 82% for the control (p<0.001)
Toumpoulis et al [14]	1992-2002	Freedom from all cause mortality in patients in whom DSWI developed at 1 year, 5 years, and 10 years after the operation was 66.2%, 50.8%, and 40.6% respectively, compared with 87.2%, 72.8%, and 54.3% in patients without DSWI (p=0.0007)
Risnes et al [15]	1989-2000	The 10-year, long-term survival for patients with mediastinitis was 49.5%, compared with 71.0% in non-mediastinitis patients (p<0.01)
Sjoegren et al [18]	1999-2004	The actuarial survival at 1 year, 3 years, and 5 years was 92.9% , 89.2%, and 89.2% for patients with mediastinitis and 96.5%, 92.1%, and 86.9 for those without mediastinitis(p=0. 578)
Sachithanandan et al [22]	2001-2005	Unadjusted freedom from all-cause mortality in patients with DSWI at 1 year, 2 years, and 3 years after surgery was 78.6 ± 4.8% (95% CI 69–88.2%), 75.6 ± 5.0% (95% CI 65.6–85.6%) and 69.4 ± 5.8% (95% CI 57.8–81%) respectively compared with 92.8 ± –0.4% (95% CI 92.4–93.2%), 90.7 ± 0.5% (95% CI 90.2–91.2%) and 87.7 ± 0.6% (95% CI 87.1–88.3%) for patients without DSWI (p < 0.001)
Bailot et [46]	1992-2007	Survival in patients with DSWI showed freedom from all-cause mortality at 1, 5 and 10 years to be, respectively, 91.8%, 80.4% and 61.3% compared with 94.0%, 85.5% and 70.2%, respectively, for patients (p = 0.01). Adjusted survival for patients with DSWI treated with NPWT was 92.8%, 89.8% and 88.0%, respectively, at 1, 2 and 3 years, compared with 83.0%, 76.4% and 61.3%, respectively, for patients with DSWI treated conventionaly(p = 0.02)

Table 3. Analyses of compared mid-term and long-term survival of patients with DSWI with non-DSWI patients

Patients who develop DSWI are 2.5 to 3 times more expensive to manage compared with patients who have an uncomplicated post-operative course [6,11]. The first calculation of cost originated from the Loop et al paper, published in the late 1980's, and found a 2.8 times increase in cost [6]. Patients who died of DSWI consequences consumed 60,500 USD more, making the total cost of these patients approximately 80,000 USD compared with 11,000 USD an uncomplicated CABG patient cost, as showed by Hollenbeak et al [11]. Recent data from Germany showed a doubling in cost (36,261 vs. 13,356 EUR, p<0.001) for DSWI patients [49], while Ennker et al calculated a 9,000 EUR increase in cost on average for any DSWI case [50]. The majority of the increased cost is spent on repeat surgical and ICU service, and extension of in-hospital stay [11,51,52]. In looking for cost-effectiveness of treatment strategies, NPWT does not seem to be a more expensive treatment in comparison with the conventional therapy for DSWI, as calculated in the Swedish healthcare system by Mokhari et al [52]. Atkins et al reported lower NPWT costs than Medicare charges for conventional therapy (152,000 vs. 300,000 USD) of DSWI [53].

5. Strategies preventing DSWI

As mentioned previously, diabetes mellitus is a strong independent risk factor for development of DSWI, and concomitant obesity doubles the risk of further infection [24]. Unfortunately, both risk factors are difficult to modify. Zerr et al showed that a continuous insulin infusion started immediately after surgery to maintain a serum glucose level of 150-200mg/dl (8-11 mmol/l) led to a significant decrease in the incidence of DSWI in diabetics (2.4% to 1.5%, p < 0.02) compared with subcutaneously administered insulin [54]. A tight glycemic control protocol appears beneficial from the Portland group experience, nevertheless, decreasing serum glucose below 100mg/dl (6 mmol/l) did not bring any additional impact on DSWI rate, and was associated with a higher risk of stroke or death [55].

It has been demonstrated many times that antibiotic prophylaxis effectively prevents sternal wound infection [56]. As Staphylococcal stains are a major causative pathogen, beta-lactam antiobiotics are recommended for prophylaxis, particularly first or second generation cephalosporins [57]. The use of glycopeptides, which are highly effective against MRSA, has not been linked with a reduction in sternal wound infection rates compared to standard prophylaxis, with one study suggesting higher SSI's rate (3.7 vs. 1.3%, p<0.05) when vancomycin prophylaxis was chosen [58]. Local application of a gentamicin soaked-collagen sponge between the sternal lamella was suggested to reduce all SWI's, particularly DSWI. Friberg et al reported a significant reduction in SWI's (3.7 vs. 9%, p<0.001), and also DSWI (1.5 vs. 3.3%, p<0.003) [59,60], however, further randomized controlled trials and meta-analyses did not confirm a benefit of using a gentamicin sponge for DSWI prevention as well as a recently published meta-analysis [61,62]. Although SA caused DSWI might be reduced by locally applied gentamicin, primarily gentamicin-resistant strains such a CONS may overgrow [62].

Another prophylactic issue is patient decontamination before surgery. As Staphylococci colonization is seen in a majority of DSWI, skin and nasopharyngeal decontamination became popular [38,39]. The use of chlorhexidine for skin care before surgery showed a significant reduction in the microbial count including SA [63]. In comparison to general surgery where reduction of SSI's due to skin decontamination was confirmed [64], data for cardiac surgery is lacking, nevertheless, protocols involving chlorhexidine or a different skin cleanser are already widely accepted. Locally applied ointment containing mupirocin is 80 to 90% effective in eradicating all types of SA from the nasopharyngeal mucosa [65]. Cimochowski et al reported about the efficacy of this practice on reducing DSWI rates from 2.7% to 0.9% [66]. A randomized controlled trial published by Konvalinka et al did not confirm a reduced DSWI rate from the use of nasal mupirocin ointment (0.8 vs. 0.8%) [67].

The surgical technique in performing median sternotomy and its closure certainly influences the risk of DSWI. Careful handling of skin and pre-sternal soft tissue, mid-lined sternal incision and avoidance of bone wax are essential, in addition to keeping scrub protocol, checking for glove injury, changing gloves after sternotomy and after sternal wiring, and leaving the closed wound primarily covered for at least 48 hours [68].

It has been proposed that the method of IMA harvesting affects the incidence of DSWI, particularly when both IMA (BIMA's) are demanded for revascularization [7,8,10,27,28]. A recent meta-analysis published by Saso et al showed a reduced risk of SWI's once IMA or BIMA's were harvested in a skeletonized fashion compared with a pedicled graft. The risk was reduced both in the non-diabetic (2.96% vs. 11.7%) and diabetic populations (2.4% vs. 14.2%) [69]. Besides harvesting methods of BIMA's in diabetics, as was mentioned above, tight long-term glycemic control influenced the risk of DSWI. A hemoglobin A1c (HbA1c) $\geq 7\%$ had a higher incidence of DSWI compared with patients who had a HbA1c $<7\%$ (5.0% vs. 1.4%, P = 0.014). A 31% increased risk of DSWI (OR = 1.31, 95% CI 1.16-1.49, P < 0.001) was seen by Halkos et al [26]. Even through diabetic patients may have a comparable risk of developing DSWI when IMA in skeletonized fashion is taken down, the BIMA's harvesting need is to be considered carefully because additional risk factors such an obesity and COPD are commonly presented in this cohort [24,70].

The crucial point in preventing DSWI is achievement of stable sternal approximation. Standard sternal wire cerclage, if performed well, is fast, easy and effective [71]. Facing poor sternal quality, sternal fracture, or increased traction forces in obese or COPD patients, some modifications of this technique were proposed. Parasternal wire reinforcement, described originally by Robicsek and modified by Sharma, proved to reduce the risk of sternal wound complications [72,73]. Friberg et al reported that the use of more than 6 or 7 simple wires may also reduce DSWI rates (0.4% vs. 4.2%, p=0.001) [74]. Recently, a large multicenter prospective study conducted by Schimmer et al comparing the Robicsek technique with standard cerclage failed to reduce the risk of SWI and sternal dehiscence [75]. Primary plating, mirroring the experience in maxillofacial surgery, was proposed for patients at high risk of sternal non-union [76]. Plates could be anchored only into the sternal bone (SternaLock system™,Biomet Microfixation Inc, Jacksonville, US) or into the ribs (Titanium Sternal Fixation system™, Syntes, Switzeland). Raman et al reported better chest bone healing after primary plating than rewiring at 6-month follow up (70 vs. 24%, p=0.003) and lower pain scores, with no difference in SWI rates [77]. Others systems are used for sternal approximation including, thermoreactive nitinol clips

(Flexigrip™, Praesidia SRL, Bologna, Italy), titanium locked staples (Sternal Talon™, KLS Martin Group, US), and Poly-Ether-Ether-Ketone tapes (Sternal ZipFix system™, Syntes, Switzeland), all designed for parasteral fixation. Negri et al reported a significant reduction of mechanical dehiscence (2.8% vs. 0.2%, p=0.002), but the same risk of DSWI (1.2% vs. 2.4%) when thermoactive clips were compared with standard wire cerclage [78]. Snyder et al reported 5 years of experience with the SternaLock system™ for primary plating in high risk patients. Superiority of plate over wires was seen in the incidence of early presentation (<30 days) of SWI (0% vs. 12%, p<0.06) and shorter in-hospital stay (7 vs. 8 days, p=0.02) [79]. A pilot study published by Bennett-Guerrero et al showed insignificantly higher spirometry volume in the SternalTalon™ arm (67% ± 32%) versus the wire arm (58% ± 24%). Use of the Talon was associated with decreased use of opiates (21.3 ± 11.8 vs. 25.4 ± 21.6 mg, P = 0.44), duration of mechanical ventilation (0.5 vs. 1.0 days, P = 0.24) and hospital length of stay (4.5 ± 3.2 vs. 5.3 ± 4.0 days, P = 0.40) [80].

A promising method to reduce SSI seems to be the application of NPWT on surgically closed sternal wounds. A commercially available system (Prevena® Incision Management System, KCI, St. Antonio, USA) is used, with skin preservation through a semipermeable membrane that has contact with foam, and one proposal pump system with reservoir is added [81]. Limited clinical experience has shown a decreased risk of wound hematoma, seroma and SSI [82]. Other positive effects from wound application of NPWT might include promotion of microvascular flow and decreased tissue edema and myofibroblast activation [83]. Colli and Atkins et al reported no wound healing complications in patients at high risk for sternal wound infections after cardiac surgery, but both studies were retrospective and done on smaller cohort of patients, 10 and 57, respectively [84,85].

6. Treatment strategies for DSWI

Even though treatment of DSWI has considerably evolved, a generally accepted treatment strategy remains controversial. Robicsek postulated three valid principles addressing this issue: first, that the infectious process should be brought under control within the shortest possible time, secondly, that adequate debridement and drainage of the infected area should occur, and third that sternal stability should be assured [86]. Until the 1960s, patients suffering from DSWI were treated conservatively with antibiotic therapy, limited drainage, or exposure of the sternotomy wound until closure with granulation tissue occurred [87]. Mortality rates then reached over 50% and survivors' quality of life was limited due to significant morbidity [87]. In 1964, Shumacker and Mandelbaum reported their experience with single-stage technique of wound debridement, primary sternal re-wiring and continuous antibiotic irrigation [88]. Their original method was consequently modified in terms of the type of antibiotic or antiseptic solution used including its amount, or the setting of indwelling drains for irrigation and suction [89-90]. Closed chest drainage became widely used with reported mortality from DSWI ranging from 4.8% to 28%, with an associated risk of primary therapy failure ranging from 12.5% to 48% [89,90-92]. Lee et al proposed in 1976 the use of an omental flap for covering infected sternotomy wounds [93]. Vital greater omentum was turned into the chest cavity following sternal debridement. It was suggested that well-vascularized omentum fulfills dead spaces, ensures high antibiotic levels, and yielded angiogenic and absorptive capacity [13,93]. Jurkiewicz et al first reported the use of muscle flaps, preferably the pectoralis flap, and radical sternal debridement in the treatment of DSWI in 1980 [94]. Consequently, 20-years of experience in the Emory group with 409 patients showed 8.1% in-hospital mortality and 5.1% primary therapy failure. 87.1% of procedures were done in single-stage fashion; the pectoralis major was used in 76.6%, rectus abdominis in 19.4%, and omentum in 2.2% [95]. This approach has received many modifications regarding the timing of wound closure, choice of flap, and type of advancement, with reported mortality ranging from 0% to 19% [96,97]. Comparing the omental to the pectoralis flap, Milano et al reported that the omental flap had lower mortality (4.8% vs. 10.5%, p<0.05), early wound related complications (9.5% vs. 27.7%, p<0.001), and in-hospital stay (10.7 vs. 18.8%, p<0.05) [98]. El Oakley and Wright suggested classification of DSWI based on the time of presentation, presence of risk factors such as obesity, diabetes or immunosuppressive therapy, and number of failed therapeutic attempts in 1996 (Table 3) [99]. The identification of five subtypes of DSWI seemed to be a relevant tool for choice of therapeutic method and patient prognosis. Adjusted to the El Oakley and Wright classification, closed chest irrigation has comparable mortality data for type I and II DSWI compared with radical sternal resection and concomitant flap, but with lower flap-related associated morbidity [100-102]. Ringelman et al noted that at 48 month follow-up, 51% of patients had pain or discomfort, 44% had numbness, 42% complained of sternal instability, and 33% claimed to have shoulder weakness, when pectoral flap was used for reconstruction [103]. Closed chest irrigation carries a higher rate of therapy failure when used for type III, and particularly type IV and V El Oakley and Wright classification [104-107]. Thus, these patients might have benefit from more radical sternal debridement and employment of well-vascular-ized tissue to replenish residual defects. Flap-related morbidity may be addressed with less invasive techniques such as a laparoscopic greater omentum harvesting [108]. Atkins et al recently reported on the influence of sternal repair choice (pectoral, omental flap, or secondary closure) on long-term survival [109].

There is limited data evaluating hyperbaric oxygen (HBO) therapy in the treatment of SWI, despite theoretical advantages, availability of HTO close to the cardiac surgical unit impedes its routine use [110]. Siondalski et al reported successful healing of 55 DSWI patients with no mortality, nevertheless therapy required 20-40 HBO sessions after surgical revision. HTO was taken as an adjunct therapy to perform radical debridement and muscle flap [111].

Class	Description of DSWI
Type I	Mediastinitis presenting within 2 weeks after operation in the absence of risk factors
Type II	Mediastinitis presenting at 2 to 6 weeks after operation in the absence of risk factors
Type IIIA	Mediastinitis type I in the presence of one or more risk factors
Type IIIB	Mediastinitis type II in the presence of one or more risk factors
Type IVA	Mediastinitis type I, II, or III after one failed therapeutic trial

Class	Description of DSWI
Type IVB	Mediastinitis type I, II, or III after more than one failed therapeutic trial
Type V	Mediastinitis presenting for the first time more than 6 weeks after operation
Accepted risk factors: diabetes, obesity, immunosupressive therapy intake	

Table 4. El Oakley and Wright classification of DSWI (modified from El Oakley et[99])

In 1997, Obdeijin et al described the first application of NPWT for treatment of DSWI in 3 consecutive patients [112]. They found that physical therapy contracted the wound, provided sufficient chest stability, and allowed patients to be extubated. Catarino et al reported the first retrospective comparison between NPWT and closed chest irrigation in 2000. In comparing 9 versus 10 patients, they found superiority of NPWT in length of in-hospital stay (15 vs. 40.5 days, p=0.02) and therapy failure (0 vs. 5, p=0.03) [113]. Furthermore, Gustafsson et al and Fleck et al, from the two most active European centers (Lund and Vienna), reported similar in-hospital and 30-day or 90-day mortality of DSWI patients, with 60% of all cases having class III according to El Oakley and Wright [114,115]. Consequently, the Lund group reported survival data from 1,3, and 5 year follow-up which showed comparable survival (92.9%, 89%, 89%) with patients without DSWI after CABG (96%, 92%, 86%) and showed potential survival benefit of NPWT therapy unlike data known from conventional therapy [18]. Recently published data from a larger group of patients showed 1.1-5.4% mortality at 30 days and 8-15% 1 year mortality with a 2 to 6% risk of primary therapy failure [116-119]. The mean length of application of NPWT was 8 to 14 days with a mean number of 4 to 6 dressing changes [116-119]. The amount of dressing used by centers has only minor variability in first-line application protocol, with the only differences reported being the materials used for interface dressing and the timing of wound closure [116-119]. It was suggested that low C-reactive protein level (<50 mg/l) might be a good indicator for timing of wound closure [120]. Since the introduction of NPWT, its comparison with conventional therapy, closed chest irrigation or sternal resection and flap have been studied. So far, we have data only from retrospective comparative studies, with the compared arms being heterogeneous in number of patients, time periods and type of DSWI based on El Oakley classification. It was suggested that NPWT positively influenced the risk of primary therapy failure and survival of patients at short and long-term follow-up [18,46,121-138]. Outcomes of NPWT are DSWI causative pathogen independent, even comparing therapeutic response to MRSA and MSSA caused DSWI [139]. From multivariable analyses, obesity, renal failure and sepsis were calculated as independent risk factors of NPWT failure [128,129]. Results of comparative studies and published meta-analyses are shown in Table 5.

Authors	Follow-up	Patients cohort	Endpoints	Results
Catarino et al [113]	Retrospective	11 pts NPWT vs. 9 pts closed irrigation	In-hospital stay, primary therapy failure	NPWT linked with shorter in-hospital stay (15 vs. 40.5 days, p=0.02) and lower therapy failure (0 vs. 5%, p=0.03) than closed irrigation

Authors	Follow-up	Patients 'cohort	Endpoints	Results
Berg et al [121]	Retrospective	31 pts NPWT vs. 29 pts closed irrigation	Primary therapy failure, in-hospital stay and mortality	NPWT group had a lower risk of therapy failure (52 vs. 16%, p<0.05) and in-hospital stay (22 vs. 26 days, p<0.05), with comparable in-hospital mortality (6,9 vs. 6,6%, NS) to closed irrigation
Doss et al [122]	Retrospective	22 pts NPWT vs. 22 closed irrigation	Primary therapy failure, in-hospital stay and mortality	NPWT group had shorter overall length of therapy (17.2±5.8 vs. 22.9±10.8 days, p=0.01) and in-hospital stay (27.9±6.6 vs. 33.0±11.0 dnů, p=0.03), with comparable mortality (5 vs. 5%, NS) to closed irrigation
Song et al [123]	Retrospective	17 pts NPWT vs. 18 pts open packing	Primary therapy failure, number of dressing changes, in-hospital stay and mortality	NPWT associated with shorter length of therapy (6.2 vs. 8.5 days, p<0,05), lower number of dresssing changes (3±2.5 vs. 17±8.6 , p<0.01), and comparable in-hospital mortality (11 vs. 6%, NS)
Luckraz et al [124]	Retrospective	27 pts NPWT vs. 13 pts closed irrigation	Primary therapy failure, in-hospital mortality, and cost of therapy	NPWT linked with lower therapeutic failure rate (15 vs. 30.7%, p<0.05), in-hospital mortality (7.5% vs. 18.5%, p<0.05) and overall cost of therapy (16 400 vs. 20 000 USD) compared with closed irrigation
Fuchs et al [125]	Retrospective	35 pts NPWT vs. 33 pts open packing	Lenght to achieve sterile woud, length of therapy, in-hospital stay, and 1-year survival	NPWT led to faster bacterial decontamination of wounds (16 vs. 26 days, p<0.01), shorter length of therapy (21 vs. 28 days, p<0.01) and in-hospital stay (25 vs. 34 days, p<0.01) and better 1-year survival (97.1 vs. 74.7%, p<0,05) compared with open packing
Sjoegren at el [126]	Retrospective	61 pts NPWT vs. 40 closed irrigation/ open packing	Therapy failure, 1- and 5-year mortality	NPWT had lower risk of therapy failure (0 vs. 15%,p<0.01), 90 day mortality (0 vs. 15%, p<0,01), and 1- and 5-year survival (93 vs. 82%, 83 vs. 59%, p<0.05) against conventional therapy
Immer et al [127]	Retrospective	38 pts NPWT vs. 17 sternectomy and flap	In-hospital stay and in-hospital mortality, quality of life	NPWT led to shorter in-hospital stay (51.5±20.8 vs. 70.7±28.8 dnů, p<0.05), non-significantly lower in-hospital mortality (5.3 vs 11.8, NS) and better quality of life based on questionnaire SF-36 compared with sternectomy and flap

Authors	Follow-up	Patients ´cohort	Endpoints	Results
Segers [128]	Retrospective	29 pts NPWT vs. 34 pts closed irrigation	Therapy failure, in-hospital, and 1-year mortality	NPWT decreased primary therapy failure (27.6 vs. 58.9%, p<0.05), with comparable 30 day (3,5 vs. 2,9%, NS)and 1-year mortality (31.0 vs. 23.5%, NS) to closed irrigation
Bailot et al [46]	Retrospektive conventional and prospective for NPWT	125 pts NPWT vs. 24 pts. open packing	In-hospital mortality and 1-,5-, and 10 years survival	Lower mortality in NPWT group (4.8 vs. 14.1%, p=0.01), but insignificantly better 1,5, and 10 year survival(92.8 vs. 83.0%, 89.8 vs. 76.4%, 88.0 vs. 61.3%, NS)
Petzina et al [129]	Retrospective	69 pts NPWT vs. 49 closed irrigation	Primary therapy failure, in-hospital stay and mortality	NPWT associated with lower therapeutic failure (2.9% vs.18.3% p<0.05) and in-hospital mortality (5.8% vs. 24.5% p<0.05), but comparable in-hospital stay (38 vs. 41 days, NS) with closed Irrigation
Simek et al [130]	Retrospective for conventional and propective pro NPWT	38 pts withNPWT vs. 28 pts closed irrigation	Primary therapy failure, in-hospital stay, in-hospital, and 1 year mortality	NPWT had lower failure of primary therapy (5.8 vs. 39.2%, p<0.05), ICU stay (209.6±33.3 vs. 516.1±449.5 hours, p<0.01),and in-hospital (5.8 vs. 21.4%, p<0.05) and 1-year mortality (14.7 vs 39.2%, p<0.05), but comparable in-hospital stay (40.2±16.3 vs. 48.8±29.2, NS) with closed irrigation.
De Feo et al [131]	Retrospective	74 pts NPWT vs. 83 pts closed irrigation	Primary therapy failure, in-hospital stay and mortality	NPWT group with lower risk of therapy failure (1.4 vs. 16.9%, p<0.001), shorter in-hospital stay (23.3±9 vs. 3.0.5±3, p<0,05), and lower in-hospital mortality (1.4 vs. 3,6 %, p<0,.05) compared with closed irrigation
Assman et al [132]	Retrospective	82 pts NPWT vs. 38 closed irrigation	In-hospital stay and mortality	NPWT patients had shorter in-hospital stay (45.6 ± 18.5 vs. 55.2 ± 23.6 dnů, p<0.05), and lower in-hospital mortality (14.6 vs. 32.4 %, p<0.05)
Vos et al [133]	Retrospective	89 pts NPWT vs. 24 open packing	In-ICU and hospital stay and mortality	NPWT led to shorter ICU stay (6.8±14.4 vs. 18.5±21.0 dnů, p<0.01), in-hospital stay (74.4±61.2 vs. 69.1±62.7 days, p<0.01), and lower in-hospital mortality (12.4 vs. 41.7%, p<0.01)
Deniz et al [134]	Retrospective	47 pts NPWT vs. 43 closed irrigation	Primary therapy failure, in-hospital stay and 1-, 3 years mortality	NPWT had insignificantly lower rate of primary therapy failure (2.1% vs. 4.7%, NS) and shorter in-hospital stay (18±9 vs. 24±10 days, NS), 90 days mortality significantly lower (8.5 vs. 23.2%, p<0.05) and better 1-, and 3-year

Authors	Follow-up	Patients 'cohort	Endpoints	Results
				survival (91.5% vs.76.7%, p<0,05, 87.2 vs 69.8%, P<0.05)
Fleck et al [135]	Retrospective	326 pts NPWT vs. 198 closed irrigation/ open packing	Primary therapy failure, in-hospital mortality	NPWT was associated with lower primary therapy failure (8.5% vs. 34% p<0.001), and in-hospital mortality (3.6% vs. 10%, p<0.05)
Sjoegren at el [18]	Meta-analysis	12 papers focused on comparison of NPWT with conventional therapy	Primary therapy failure, in-hospital stay and mortality	NPWT associated with lower primary therapy failure, shorter in-hospital stay, and lower in-hospital and 1-year mortality
Raja et al [136]	Meta-analysis	13 papers focused on comparison of NPWT with conventional therapy	Primary therapy failure, in-hospital stay and mortality	NPWT seemed to be effective at high-risk DSWI patients, but weak evidence for routine first-line application in DSWI
Schimmer et al [137]	Meta-analysis	15 papers focused on comparison of NPWT with conventional therapy	Primary therapy failure, in-hospital stay and mortality, evaluation of German hearts centers protocols	NPWT is associated with lower therapeutic failure, and in-hospital mortality. Routinely applied as first-line treatment in 35% of German heart centers
Damiani G et al [138]	Meta-analysis	6 papers focused on comparison of NPWT with conventional therapy and chest reconstruction options	Primary therapy failure, in-hospital stay and mortality	NPWT prone to have shorter in-hospital stay and lower mortality

Table 5. Analyses and Meta-analyse of comparison NPWT with conventional therapy

Addressing specific complications of DSWI, it is seen that NPWT does not increase the risk of late infection recurrence. Reported rates of chronic fistulas after conventional therapy and NPWT were comparable between 8-12% [18,130,134,140,41], and long-term survival of these patients is negatively affected [140,142]. CONS was identified as a pathogen with a higher risk of recurrence; its low virulence, ability to create biofilm on metallic materials and inherent low sensitivity against prophylactically administrated antibiotics limit its eradication [41,143].

With the rise in use of NPWT came an increased number of reported serious bleeding complications [144,145]. The risk of heart injury, particularly the right ventricle, bypass grafts or great vessels is well known from conventionally treated patients. Infectious erosion, displacement of heart structures towards sternal margins, or tractions of fibrosis adhesion were identified as potential mechanism of injury [146]. The incidence of these complications by conventional therapy was found to be between 2-14.8% [147-149], with data from a larger group of NPWT treated patients showing 2 to 5%, thus NPWT does not seem to increase the incidence of serious complications [116,118,127,130,146,150]. Mortality from these complications varies between 25 to 70%, with emergency surgery as well as proper covering of mediastinal structures with interface dressing being crucial for management [146-148,150]. Several layers of paraffin gauze or silicone mesh are usually put below sternal margins on the heart and grafts. Development towards more suitable material, particularly rigid barrier for mediastinal protection is in progress, including mediastinal protection and preserved drainage ability of therapy [151].

7. Reconstruction of sternal bone defect after DSWI in cardiac surgery

Wire re-cerclage was a commonly used method for addressing sternal approximation in patients with sternal dehiscence after DSWI [72,86,102]. The quality of residual sternal bone or its loss makes re-cerclage troublesome or even risky for achieving sternal stability. The occurrence of extensive adhesions below the sternum in DSWI patients increases the risk of damage to the right ventricle and bypass grafts when peri-, trans- and parasternal wiring techniques are used [72,99,100]. Today, stable osteosynthesis of the sternum, particularly using transverse plates, has become a method of treatment of post-DSWI sternal dehiscence [76]. Voss at el reported an institutional experience with Titanium Sternal Fixation system™ plates for sternal non-union in 15 patients, in which four patients had more than two previous attempts to stabilize the chest with some modification of wire re-cerclage, and four patients were treated for DSWI with NPWT prior to plating. All patients were successfully stabilized and healed, with one patient from the DSWI group experiencing a late infection recurrence and one dying from a complication not related to plating [152]. Larger experience with the same plate system has been reported by Baillot et al in a group of 92 patients after DSWI [46]. They achieved chest stabilization in all cases, with 9 patients (9.8%) undergoing further procedure for late infection recurrence including removal of the plate with no impact on sternal stability [153]. Chest stability after a healed DSWI improves respiratory function, augments wound healing processes, shortens in-hospital stay, and improves patient quality [46,72,80]. Plating seems to be an effective method of chest wall stabilization, but may fail in cases of massive loss of chest bone tissue. In these cases, the bone residue does not allow sufficient anchoring for the plates or there is a large bone tissue gap. Shear forces may loosen screws and threaten stability. Persistent pain and respiratory discomfort were also reported in this case [154]. A conventional surgical approach to manage the large residual bone defect leaves the sternotomy wound unstable and employs the greater omentum or a muscle flap to fulfill any dead spaces [93,95,99,103]. This approach resulted in sternal instability and flap-related morbidity even when wounds were well-healed [154]. Some case reports have included the use of an autologous bone iliac crest graft or allogenous fibula graft to supply residual bone defects after DSWI [155,156]. Marulli reported the first use of an allogenous sternocostal bone graft for sternal reconstruction after chondrosarcoma removal [157]. Consequently, Dell'amore et al described four patients who were managed with the same technique with no wound healing complications and preserved chest wall stability [158]. The same authors proposed this technique for major post-DSWI defects, and [159] Kalab et al described the possibility of using an allogenous calva bone graft to address this issue. Allogenous bony grafts being fixed with transverse plates in mentioned cases [158-160]. Bone allograft usage for transplantation is under law restriction of local governments and European Association of Tissue Banks [161,162].

8. Options in soft tissue defects reconstruction after DSWI in cardiac surgery

There are a broad range of possibilities for managing sternal soft tissue defects caused by DSWI. In the case of minor defects, a direct suture with tissue undermining can be effective. In wide dehiscence, some type of flap transfer is needed and excessive bone and soft tissue loss are dependent on close co-operation between the cardiac and reconstructive surgeons. There are two crucial conditions influencing the reconstructive strategy. The first condition is the size of the defect, while the second is the vascular network, which would optimally remain uncompromised after primary surgery or previously failed reconstructions. Although various flaps and their modifications have been proposed, none have been found to be a reconstructive option for all defects [97,163,164], therefore Greig et al suggested a simple classification system to address the choice of flap based on the size and location of the post-sternotomy defect (Table 6) [165]. It is not possible, however, to follow this classification system because various factors and conditions influencing the result must be taken into the account.

Wound type	Site of sternal wound	Recommended flap for reconstruction
Type A	Upper half sternum	Pectoralis major
Type B	Lower half sternum	Combined pectoralis major and rectus abdominis bipedicled flap
Type C	Whole sternum	Combined pectoralis major and rectus abdominis bipedicled flap

Table 6. Classification of sternal wounds according to anatomical site (modified from Greig et al [165])

In 1976, Lee et al were the first to report on the use of a pedicled greater omentum to fulfill the large defect after total sternectomy [93]. In 1980, Jurkiewicz et al introduced the bilateral pectoralis turnover flap for the same indication. Although various muscle flaps, along with their modifications have been reported, there is still debate about using muscular versus cutaneous or fasciocutaneous flaps to cover difficult defects. It has been presumed that muscular flaps carry richer vascular networks, thus bringing a better blood supply to the defect, along with a higher antibiotic concentration. Recent studies, however, did not support this hypothesis and suggested that muscle flaps have no particular advantage over fasciocutaneous flaps in terms of improving vascularity and eradicating infection [166,167]. Nevertheless, there is still a reasonable argument for muscular flaps as additional muscle brings enough tissue for planed reconstruction.

8.1. The pectoralis major flap

The pectoralis major provides many qualities that make it a suitable flap choice for covering sternal defects including close proximity to the sternotomy, triple blood supply (the thoracoacromial artery, perforating branches of the internal thoracic artery and the lateral thoracic artery), and versatility of the flap as either the thoracoacromial or internal thoracic artery vascular axis may be used separately to nourish the flap [168]. Netcher et al did not show an adverse influence of the pectoral muscle transposition on pulmonary function [169], moreover, pain and loss of strength appeared to be related more to sternal instability rather than to the muscle transposition. Additionally, Cohen et al reported an improvement of spirometric parameters (forced vital capacity and standardized forced expiratory volume in 1 second) before and after pectoral flap transfer, thus supporting the crucial role of the flap in chest stabilization [170].

8.1.1. Pectoral muscle advancement flap

The pectoral muscle advancement flap is based on the thoracoacromial pedicle and is considered to be the best muscular reconstructive option in this area due to its technical simplicity, versatility, and low risk of flap loss (<3%). There is, however, some risk of skin island necrosis or partial necrosis (≈30%) [171, 172]. Dissection and elevation of the flap begins along the median line of the costal grid until reaching the relatively avascular plane under the muscle. Undermining then proceeds by blunt dissection laterally as necessary to achieve approximation of the bilateral flaps at the median line without tension. The thoracoacromial vascular pedicle is visible at the dorsal plane of the muscle. The humeral and clavicular insertion of the muscle can be released if needed. If the distal portion of the sternum is exposed, dissection continues distally under the anterior sheet of the rectus abdominis which then becomes part of the flap [164]. Though the flap is elevated mostly in a myocutaneous fashion [73,163,164,173,174], Brutus et al reported on the use of a pectoral muscle flap released from skin for covering the entire sternal defect [175]. Completely dissected and freed from all of its origins, the pectoral muscle was advanced medially on the skeletonized vascular pedicle to cover the full length of the sternal defect. Separating the skin from the muscle can jeopardize the cutaneous blood supply and increase risk of skin necrosis. This technique included the release of humeral insertion from a short skin counter incision [175].

If the defect is wide, it may be difficult to achieve tension-free suturing in the midline. A modification of the advancement flap with a skin relaxing incision has been reported [176]. Majure et al proposed shifting the skin island over the pectoralis muscle in the V-Y manner to cover the entire sternotomy defect, but this method requires secondary skin grafting from an island donor site [177]. This technique was adopted and modified by Molitor et al [178]. The skin island is dissected, while the underlying muscle fascia and pectoralis major are elevated and completely released from their insertions to the humerus, sternocostal junctions and abdominal muscles. The thoracoacromial vessels are visualized and the clavicular insertion of the muscle is released to achieve comfortable advancement of the flap to the defect. The secondary defect in the lateral thoracic wall is then sutured in the V-Y manner and no skin graft is needed [178].

Finally, the pectoralis major musculocutaneous flap can be mobilized in a rotational manner when the skin-muscle flap is elevated based on the thoracoacromial pedicle and is rotated to the defect [179].

8.1.2. Pectoral muscle turnover flap

This flap is based on perforators of the internal mammary artery. Once the skin is elevated off of the anterior pectoralis fascia, the distal rib, proximal clavicular origin and humeral insertion of the muscle are divided. Then, the thoracoacromial pedicle is dissected and ligated, and the pectoralis major is elevated from lateral to medial until the perforating vessels from the internal thoracic artery are identified, and the muscle is then turned into the defect. To gain additional width of the narrowing humeral portion of the flap, fascial release incisions along the direction of the muscle fibers can be done. By this maneuver an average increase in flap width of 5.8 cm can be obtained [181]. Usually bilateral turnover muscle flaps are used [94,95]. The disadvantages of this flap include limitations in the distal parts of the sternum, need for wide skin undermining, dependence on an intact internal mammary artery, and an unfavorable aesthetic consequence including a missing anterior axillary line and parasternal subcutaneous tissue bulkiness [95].

8.2. The rectus abdominis flap

This flap was first used in cardiac surgery by Jurkiewicz in the case of a pectoral turnover flap failing to cover the entire defect [94,95]. To cover the sternal defect, the rectus abdominis flap is used exclusively as a pedicled flap based on the superior epigastric artery [182]. Because this artery is the terminal branch of the internal thoracic artery, the flap cannot be used if the ipsilateral internal thoracic artery was used for bypass grafting. The functional consequences of using the rectus abdominis to reconstruct sternal defects were assessed by Netscher et al [169]. They found no significant differences in abdominal wall function between the groups of patients in whom the rectus muscle was used for reconstruction and the group without sternal wound complications. There is a higher associated risk of hernia (11%) or fascial weakness (42%) as was reported [103,183]. The rectus abdominis flap may be used as a muscular flap [94,184) or as a myocutaneous island flap [171,185].

8.2.1. Rectus abdominis muscular flap

The rectus abdominis muscular flap may be dissected without the use of a skin island. The skin incision continues distally to the desired point according to the necessary flap length. The skin is undermined over the rectus fascia to expose the muscle. Then, the rectus anterior sheet is divided and the muscle is dissected and mobilized. The distal pedicle inferior epigastric vessels are ligated and divided. The muscle is then turned to the defect. The exposed muscle and pedicle is covered either by skin suture or grafting [95].

8.2.2. Rectus abdominis musculocutaneous flap

The myocutaneous flap can have a skin island oriented vertically along the used muscle (VRAM-vertical rectus abdominis muscle flap), or horizontally, as well as perpendicular to the muscle distal to the umbilicus (TRAM-transverse rectus abdominis muscle flap). The transverse orientation permits harvest of a larger skin paddle. Dissection of the VRAM starts with marking the skin island over the used muscle. The skin component should be placed medially near the umbilicus to include important periumbilical perforators. The skin island is cut and the skin overlying the muscle is undermined above the muscle fascia. Then, the rectus sheet is divided bilaterally at the edges of the muscle and the muscle is dissected and mobilized. The distal pedicle inferior epigastric vessels are ligated and divided. The flap is then turned to the defect. The TRAM is marked transversely under the umbilicus and skin island which can involve the entire area between the umbilicus and symphysis bilaterally. The flap is dissected in the similar way as the VRAM flap, but the mobilization of the skin island continues away from the muscle pedicle crossing the midline to the contralateral side [171,185]. Care must be taken to avoid pedicle compression passed through the subcutaneous tunnel to the sternal defect.

8.3. Combined pectoral muscle — Rectus abdominis muscle flap

For full length sternal defects, a combined pectoralis major and rectus abdominis flap (Pec-Rec flap) was proposed [186]. The flap is predominantly created on the left side, but can occasionally be bilateral. The skin overlying the pectoral muscle is elevated up to the mid-axillary line laterally and from the clavicle to the inferior costal line in a vertical direction. The pectoral muscle is elevated while preserving the thoracoacromial vessels. The muscle is detached from its humeral insertion and medially from one third of the clavicle. Dissection of the flap continues distally while elevating the thoracoepigastric fascial attachments from the chest wall between the pectoralis major and the rectus abdominis. Distal to the fascia, the anterior sheet of the rectus abdominis is incised medially and laterally and the muscle is mobilized from the posterior fascia. The muscular connections of the rectus abdominis to the distal ribs are detached as the last step of flap harvesting. The superior epigastric artery can be preserved or it can be divided close to the muscle if necessary for better medial transposition of the flap [186].

8.4. The latissimus dorsi muscle flap

The latissimus dorsi flap is based on a thoracodorsal artery that has not been jeopardized by previous cardiac surgery. Moreover, a large flap can be harvested (the main surface area of muscle is 105 cm^2 for women and 192 cm^2 for men) [187]. The main disadvantages of this flap include the need for a lateral decubital position during flap harvesting that can endanger patients with large sternal bone defect and sternal instability and shoulder functional limitation followed latissimus dorsi muscle harvesting. Patients who are dependent on their shoulder girdle strength, such as paralytic patients in a wheelchair or walker dependent patients, may endorse strength difficulties after muscle harvesting as well as tennis and golf players or those whose profession involves overhead tasks [187]. Up to 50% of patients may complain of localized numbness at the harvesting area [172].

Usually the muscle from the non-dominant side is used. The arc of rotation and position of the skin island is assessed and marked. The skin component is predominantly oriented perpendicular to the muscle fibers near the vertebral column, but a longitudinal course from the medial axillary line to the medial caudal dorsum is also possible. The flap is dissected using the whole muscle up to the pedicle. Thoracodorsal vessels are skeletonized and humeral muscle insertion is divided, allowing an additional 4-10 cm of flap advancement. Then the flap is transposed to the defect through a subcutaneous tunnel superficial to the pectoralis major [188,189].

8.5. Breast flap

Obese female patients with large breasts are at higher risk of sternal dehiscence due to the infero-lateral tension of the breasts, especially on the distal third of the sternotomy [72].This instability results from the greater protrusion of the lower thorax and abdomen during respiration, greater dimensions of the lower versus the upper thorax, the concentration of forces from the attachment of the ribs, and the reduced thickness of the lower sternum [72]. Therefore a special bandage, supporting bra, or other garment is used to release the tension resulting from large breasts. The technique of covering the sternal dehiscence with a bilateral pectoral muscle advancement flap with simultaneous breast reduction has been reported [190-192]. Large breasts carry an enormous amount of relatively well vascularized tissue that can potentially be used to cover the sternal defect [193,194]. The vascular supply of the breast is basically the same as the pectoral muscle. There is, however, a unique vascular network inside the breast gland, known as Würinger's septum. Uygur et al reported a method of covering a large distal sternum defect with bilateral fasciocutaneous V-Y flaps from the breasts [193]. These flaps were anatomically based on the Würinger's septum [193,195]. Another method has been suggested by Hamdi et al [196]. They performed a septum-based therapeutic mammoplasty on two patients. The principle of this technique is to reduce breast mass with harvesting of a large fasciocutaneous flap from the inferomedial part of the breast

Another possibility for utilizing the breasts to cover the sternal defect is a Cyclops' flap. In this technique the whole breast is transposed to the central or even contralateral chest defect, so that the areola is centralized. The breast flap in this case is based on the lateral and central vascular pedicles of the breast [197,198].

8.6. Omentum

The greater omentum is a well-vascularized tissue with plentiful lymphatic drainage and angiogenic activity [93,98,199]. Its size can be up to 36x46 cm and is reliable to cover large defects. It is difficult, however, to predict the flap size preoperatively because the greater omentum volume has no direct correlation with the patient's habitus [200]. The omentum can be transposed to the defect in various ways such as, pedicled on both gastroepiploic arteries for defects in the distal part of sternotomy wound or mobilized on either of the gastroepiploic vessels to cover full-length sternotomy defects [201-203]. Passing the omental flap subcutane-ously from the upper portion of the laparotomy bears up to a 21% risk of late herniation [202], thus, a better solution seems to create the transdiaphragmatical tunnel just right of the falciform ligament [204]. The risk of abdominal cavity infection is rare [205], but the traction on the gastroepiploic artery can cause motility disturbances of the stomach and duodenum [206], and one case of fatal cecum volvulus have been reported [207]. Laparoscopic harvesting seems to be promising in reduction of access complications and pain [108,208,209].

8.7. Microsurgical flaps

Microsurgical free flaps can be used to cover sternal defects in particular situations. This technique, due to its duration and technical complexity, should serve as a last treatment option. The use of the tensor fascia lata myocutaneous flap, rectus abdominis myocutaneous flap and deep inferior epigastric artery fasciocutaneous flap for this indication have been reported [210]. As a donor vessel, the thoracoacromial, internal thoracic or cervical vessels can be used. The cephalic vein attached to the thoracoacromial or cervical arteries, can be used for lengthening the donor vessel (arterio-venous loop) [210,211].

8.8. Specifics of care after flap surgery in cardiac surgery

There are special requirements for care after flap surgery. In general, it is important to protect the blood circulation within the flap, maintaining both general and local hemodynamics. Vascular spasm must be prevented by using vasodilator drugs if possible. The elevated and transposed flap usually loses most of its physiological blood and lymphatic network and is dependent only on a small part of it, so varying degrees of edema are usually present. Large swelling of the tissue compresses the capillaries and decreases the blood flow in the flap, increasing the tension on the suture. Corticosteroids are used to prevent swelling for several days in most flap surgeries unless serious contraindications are present. The flap must be kept from topical pressure, particularly in places of passing vascular pedicle and in peripheral parts of the flap because of limited vascular competence. Undoubtedly, changes in body position influence the blood supply of the flap. Furthermore, stretching of the arms causes increased tension on the medial sternal suture. In the case of the pectoral and latissimus dorsi flap, the use of muscles of the shoulder girdle should be avoided. When using the rectus abdominis flap, the abdominal wall must be relaxed and supported with bandages for several weeks to prevent hernia formation. Finally, nutritional support with enteral feeding is essential for successful healing.

9. University hospital Olomouc management of DSWI after cardiac surgery

9.1. Adopted treatment strategy for DSWI

We retrospectively analyzed our experience with treatment strategies of DSWI since February 2002, when our department was established. A total of 100 patients fulfilling CDC criteria [5] for DSWI were enrolled until September 2011 with an overall incidence of DSWI of 1.36%. The results of 28 patients (March 2002-June 2004) primarily treated with closed chest irrigation using diluted iodine solution were compared with 76 patients (September 2004 to September 2009) treated with NPWT (VAC ATS™, KCI, St. Antonio, USA). A standardized protocol for first-line application of NPWT is depicted in Figure 1. Six patients from the interim period (June to September 2004) when closed irrigation and NPWT were combined were excluded from the analysis. Both groups had comparable demographic and perioperative characteristics, however, the NPWT arm had an insignificant trend towards advanced age, higher logistic EUROSCORE, more complex primary cardiac surgery. No difference in the rate of causative agent was found, with SA and CONS identified in almost 70% of cases. Escherichia coli (5.8%) and Pseudomonas species (7.2%) as leading Gram negative strains were cultivated. The time to presentation of DSWI was insignificant between groups (17.5±15.0 vs. 13.8±16.3, p=0.55) as well as readmission for late clinical presentation of DSWI (38.6% vs. 50%, p=0.12). Although the overall length of DSWI therapy was comparable (14.3±11.9 vs. 14.9±7.9 days, p=0.82), NPWT required more dressing changes (5.4±2.3 vs. 1.8±1.2, p<0.001), but was associated with substantially lower failure of primary therapy (5.1 vs. 39.2%, p<0.01) with closed chest irrigation. In-ICU stay was significantly shorter in the NPWT group (209.6±331.3 vs. 516.1±449.5 hours, p<0.001), nevertheless, shortened in-hospital stay (40.2±16.3 vs. 48.8±29.2 days, p=0.16) was insignificant in this group. Addressing mortality, 30-day and 1-year mortality was considerably lower in the NPWT arm (3.9 vs. 21.4%, p<0.05, 15.8 vs. 39.2%, p<0.05, respectively). A Kaplan-Meier 1 year-survival analysis is shown in Figure 2. The risk of major bleeding complications was comparable between groups, with 2 patients (3.6%) from the closed chest irrigation group having erosion of venous bypass graft and right ventricle (RV), and 3 patients (3.9%) from the NPWT group, including 1 debridement-related and 2 spontaneous injuries of the RV. Employment of local and advancement flaps for covering of residual defects was higher in the NPWT groups (65.7 vs. 17.8%, p<0.01). Our experience showed that NPWT is effective in the treatment of DSWI, compared with closed chest irrigation, leading to lower failure of primary therapy, ICU stay, and better short- and mid-survival of patients. We did not prove NPWT influenced length of in-hospital stay or risk of major bleeding, however, residual defects required more complex approach to assure sternal stability and covering defects [119,130].

9.2. Sternal stabilization and management of residual bone defects

Non-complicated sternal dehiscence following DSWI that is not associated with considerable bone loss can be stabilized with transverse titanium plates (Titanium Sternal Fixation system™, Synthes, Switzerland) at our department. Plates are applied on the anterior surface of the ribcage to achieve sufficient stability of the chest wall while minimizing the risk of an iatrogenic injury to the heart. From January 2008 to September 2012 we performed 31 sternal wall reconstructions using the Titanium Sternal Fixation system™. In four cases, osteosynthesis was applied to treat a sterile mechanical dehiscence of the median sternotomy, while 27 other chest osteosyntheses were performed after DSWI when wound bed decontamination was achieved with NPWT. In the postoperative period, 2 patients (7.4%) needed to be operatively revised due to bleeding from pectoral flap advancement; in 3 cases (11.1%) the plates needed

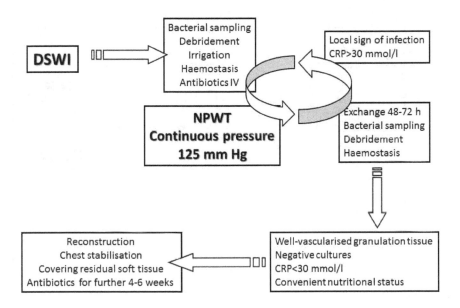

Figure 1. The first-line application protocol of NPWT for treatment of DSWI

to be removed for soft tissue healing complications post-reconstruction. Nevertheless, removal could be postponed until satisfactory healing of the sternal bones was achieved. One patient (3.7%) had to be drained for iatrogenic pneumothorax. We also retrospectively analyzed 21 patients with post-DSWI sternal dehiscence from January 2005 to January 2010, comparing 11 patients with re-cerclage wiring and 10 patients with titanium plate osteosynthesis. DSWI was managed with the same protocol of NPWT prior to reconstruction mentioned above [119]. Plating was accompanied by a lower risk of therapy failure (1% vs. 1.85%), shorter in-hospital stay (22 vs. 59%), and reduction in costs ((€8,243 vs. €33,365) (unpublished data).

In cases of minor sternal bone loss, we use an autologous bone graft harvested from the patient ′s own iliac crest. The graft is preferably prepared as bi-cortical. There is a limit to the extent of bone tissue that can be solved through this method. Fixation of the bone graft and chest stabilization is done in the manner described above. From 2009 to 2012 we used this method in 2 patients. In both cases the wounds healed successfully and the sternal wall regained full stability. Both sternal defects represented partial loss of bone tissue from 6 to 8 cm in length.

Based on this experience, we decided to apply a novel approach for the treatment of massive bone loss after DSWI, by supplying the bone defect with an allogenous bone graft. It allows

Survival Functions

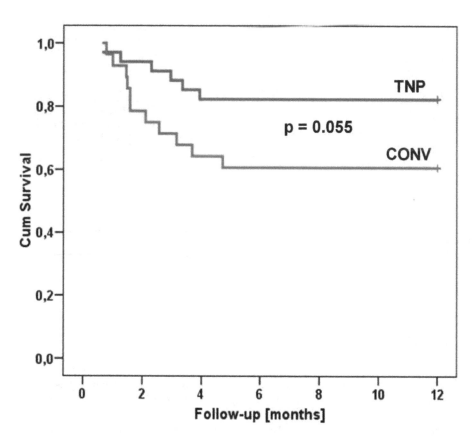

Figure 2. 1-year Kaplan-Meier survival analysis comparing NPWT with conventional therapy (CONV)

treating large sternal defects in the same way as a total or near-total sternectomy and fixed properly with titanium plate system ensures chest cage stability. An allogenous bone transplant doesn't contain any vital bone marrow cells, which eliminates difficulties in immunogenetic acceptance of the graft by a patient; it represents a biological tissue transfer, which even under conditions of maximum precautions represents a minor risk for transmission of viral or bacterial infections. An allogenous graft must meet legislative criteria from the Czech Republic and the European Association of Tissue Banks [161,162]. Prior to graft harvesting, each donor is cross-checked for registration within the National Registry for organ donation refusal. All deceased donors treated for infectious disease, sepsis, malignant tumors, or systemic and autoimmune diseases at the time of death are withdrawn from the donor list. Donor blood serum samples are tested for antibodies and HIV types 1 and 2, hepatitis B surface antigen (HbsAg), hepatitis C antibodies (anti-HCV), and HTLV I and II antibodies. Harvest of a sternal bone graft is performed under strictly sterile conditions by a team from the National Tissue Center in Brno. The graft is harvested under sterile conditions and stored in the freezer at −80°C. Prior to its clinical use, the graft is thawed at 4-6°C for 12 hours, soaked with a 1% gentamicin solution, prepared for its final shape, and stored in the freezer again at −80°C. If bacterial sampling is negative, the graft is thawed for 12 hours before transplantation, and submerged in a bath with 1% neomycin solution immediately before surgery.

Inherent surgical technique is modified by a more aggressive debridement of residual chest bone or ribs (1-2 cm safety line). Afterwards, the bone graft is adjusted to the size of the bone defect and fixed with plates anchored by self-cutting or self-drilling cortical screws. An uneven surface and tiny bone deficiency can be filled in with a spongy bone which is prepared from another graft provided by the tissue bank (femoral or tibial graft source). Residual soft tissue defect is covered with monolateral or bilateral pectoral muscle flap transfer. Within the postoperative period, it is strongly recommended to avoid excessive coughing or any rough mechanical strain on the sternal wall. Intravenous antibiotics are administered for at least three weeks after the reconstruction. Between January 2010 and September 2012, we performed six reconstructions of the sternal wall using an allogenous bone graft. We used a cadaveric sternum in four cases (Figure 3), and due to a lack of allografts, we had to use a calva bone in one patient (Figure 4) and a split femoral diaphysis in one patient. Successful healing after the reconstruction was achieved in five cases (83%), while one patient required additional treatment for partial skin necrosis. One obese female experienced flap failure and died from multiple organ failure. Follow-up of the other patients at 3, 6 and 12 months after reconstruction proved stability of the chest wall. A radio-isotope scan using technetium as a tracer of autologous leukocytes (Technetium-HMPAO) carried out at 3, 6 and 12 months after the reconstruction showed a high level of healing activity within the area of the allogenous bone implant, and further chest wall stability with allograft union was confirmed through 3D-CT evaluation done 5 to 7 months after the reconstruction (unpublished data).

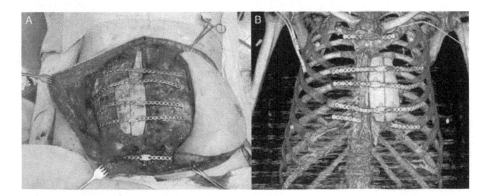

Figure 3. Cadaveric sternal allograft and its use for large residual bone defect

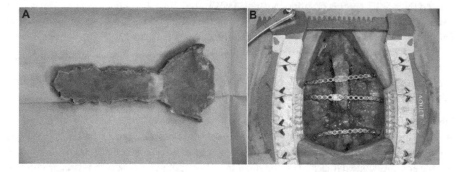

Figure 4. Cadaveric calva bone allograft in large bone defect repair and CT reconstruction showing the bone re-union

9.3. Reconstruction of residual soft tissue defects

In a group of 76 consecutive patients primarily treated with NPWT for DSWI from September 2004 to September 2011, 19 residual defects (25%) were closed by direct suture, and 57 patients (75%) underwent flap transfer to achieve reliable tension-free suture. All but 2 patients (2.7 %) underwent sternal stabilization with re-cerclage (61.8%) or transverse plates with or without bone graft (35.5%). Local fasciocutaneous advancement was used in 12 patients (21.1%), bilateral pectoralis advancement flap in 35 patients (61.2%), monolateral pectoralis flap with V-Y skin island in 7 patients (12.3%), bipedicled pectoral and rectus abdominis flap in 1 patient (1.7%), and vertical rectus abdominis flap in 2 patients (3.5%). We faced 2 flap failures (3.5%) and one whole monolateral pectoralis flap with V-Y skin island was lost due to vascular pedicle thrombosis, with 50% of the mass of the VRAM flap needing to be removed for flap necrosis. Minor healing complications requiring further local wound care were noted in 15 cases (26.3%). While the bilateral pectoralis advancement flap is a technique used by cardiac surgeons, other flaps used for covering larger residual soft tissue defects are utilized by plastic surgeon. The pectoral major flap with V-Y skin island is the first choice (Figure 5). When the defect is wide and deep, or in a female patient with large breasts, the VRAM pedicled flap is considered. If these two options fail or are not accessible, the latissimus dorsi pedicled flap is the next choice, and as a last resort, the microsurgical transfer is taken into account.

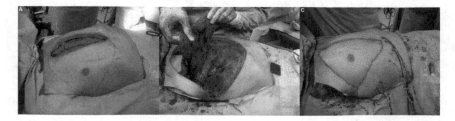

Figure 5. Technique of unilateral pectoral muscle flap advancement with V-Y skin island

10. Conclusion

DSWI remains a potentially fatal complication of cardiac surgery. Even though risk factors for development of DSWI have been identified, few are modifiable. Tight perioperative glycemic control, proper surgical technique, skeletonization of IMA grafts particularly in diabetics, and primary stable sternal approximation for high risk patients including diabetics, obese, immunosuppressed or those with COPD seem to reduce the risk of DSWI. Thanks to the unique combination of closed and open chest treatment, NPWT positively influences the survival of DSWI patients even at long-term follow-up in comparison with conventional therapy. Transverse titanium plates alone or with auto- or allograft bone allows chest cage stability irrespective to the bone mass loss. Better quality of life and lower extent of soft tissue defect might be promising for these patients who faced sternal instability and considerable flap-related morbidity some/few years ago. Plastic surgeons should be included in team planning post-DSWI sternotomy wound closure, not only called when previous closure attempt failed or residual defect seems to be extent.

Author details

Martin Šimek[1]*, Martin Molitor[1], Martin Kaláb[2], Patrick Tobbia[3] and Vladimír Lonský[1]

*Address all correspondence to: martin.simek@c-mail.cz

1 Department of Cardiac Surgery, University Hospital Olomouc, Olomouc, Czech Republic

2 Department of Plastic Surgery, University Hospital Bulovka, Prague, Czech Republic

3 Department of Medicine, Cone Health, University of North Carolina, Greensboro, NC, USA

References

[1] Dalton, M. L, Connally, S. R, & Sealy, W. C. Julian's reintroduction of Milton's operation. Ann Thorac Surg (1992). , 53, 532-533.

[2] Milton, H. Mediastinal surgery. Lancet (1897). , 1, 872-5.

[3] Julian, O. C, Lopez-belio, M, Dye, W. S, Javid, H, & Grove, W. J. The median sternal incision in intracardiac surgery with extracorporeal circulation: a general evaluation of its use in heart surgery. Surgery (1957). , 42, 753-61.

[4] Balaguer, J. M, Umakanthan, R, Leacche, M, & Byrne, J. G. Minimally invasive cardiac surgery. Curr Probl Surg. (2012). , 49, 529-49.

[5]   Mangram, A. J, Horan, T. C, Pearson, M. L, Silver, L. C, & Jarvis, W. R. The hospital
      infection control practise advisory committee. Guidelines for prevention of surgical
      site infection. Infect Control Hosp Epidemiol (2002). , 20, 247-78.

[6]   Loop, F. D, Lytle, B. W, Cosgrove, D. M, et al. Maxwell Chamberlain memorial pa-
      per. Sternal wound complications after isolated coronary artery bypass grafting: ear-
      ly and late mortality, morbidity, and cost of care. Ann Thorac Surg (1990). , 49,
      179-87.

[7]   Milano, C. A, Kesler, K, Archibald, N, Sexton, D. J, & Jones, R. H. Mediastinitis after
      coronary artery bypass graft surgery. Risk factors and long-term survival. Circula-
      tion (1995). , 92, 2245-51.

[8]   Braxton, J. H. Marrin CAS, McGrath PD, et al. Mediastinitis and long-term survival
      after coronary artery bypass graft surgery. Ann Thorac Surg (2000). , 70, 2004-7.

[9]   Eklund, A. M, Lyytikainen, O, Klemets, P, et al. Mediastinitis after more than 10,000
      cardiac surgical procedures. Ann Thorac Surg (2006). , 82, 1784-9.

[10] The Parisian Mediastinitis Study GroupRisk factors for deep sternal wound infection
      after sternotomy: a prospective, multicenter study. The Journal of Thoracic and Car-
      diovascular Surgery (1996). , 111, 1200-1207.

[11] Hollenbeak, C. S, Murphy, D. M, Koenig, S, Woodward, R. S, Dunagan, W. C, & Fras-
      er, V. J. The clinical and economic impact of deep chest surgical site infections follow-
      ing coronary artery bypass graft surgery. Chest (2000). , 118, 397-402.

[12] Filsoufi, F, Castillo, J. G, Rahmanian, P. B, et al. Epidemiology of deep sternal wound
      infection in cardiac surgery. J Cardiothorac Vasc Anesth (2009). , 23, 488-94.

[13] Tang GHL, Maganti M, Weisel RD, Borger MA. Prevention and management of deep
      sternal wound infection. Semin Thorac Cardiovasc Surg (2004). , 16, 62-9.

[14] Toumpoulis, I. K, & Anagnostopoulos, C. E. Derose JJ Jr, Swistel DG. The impact of
      deep sternal wound infection on long-term survival after coronary artery bypass
      grafting. Chest (2005). , 127, 464-71.

[15] Risnes, I, Abdelnoor, M, Almdahl, S. M, & Svennevig, J. L. Mediastinitis after coro-
      nary artery bypass grafting risk factors and long-term survival. Ann Thorac Surg
      (2010). , 89, 1502-10.

[16] Crabtree, T. D, Codd, J. E, Fraser, V. J, Bailey, M. S, & Olsen, M. A. Damiano RJ Jr.
      Multivariate analysis of risk factors for deep and superficial sternal infection after
      coronary artery bypass grafting at a tertiary care medical center. Semin Thorac Car-
      diovasc Surg. (2004). , 2004, 16-53.

[17] Fowler VG JrO'Brien SM, Muhlbaier LH, Corey GR, Ferguson TB, Peterson ED. Clini-
      cal predictors of major infections after cardiac surgery. Circulation. 200;112(9
      Suppl):I, 358-65.

[18] Sjögren, J, Malmsjö, M, Gustafsson, R, & Ingemansson, R. Poststernotomy mediastinitis: a review of conventional surgical treatments, vacuum-assisted closure therapy
and presentation of the Lund University Hospital mediastinitis algorithm.Eur J Cardiothorac Surg (2006). , 30, 898-905.

[19] Matros, E, Aranki, S. F, Bayer, L. R, et al. Reduction in incidence of deep sternal
wound infections: random or real? J Thorac Cardiovasc Surg (2010). , 139, 680-5.

[20] De Feo, M, Vicchio, M, Santè, P, Cerasuolo, F, & Nappi, G. Evolution in the treatment
of mediastinitis: single-center experience. Asian Cardiovasc Thorac Ann. (2011). , 19,
39-43.

[21] Upton, A, Roberts, S. A, Milsom, P, & Morris, A. J. Staphylococcal post- sternotomy
mediastinitis: five year audit. ANZ J Surg. (2005). , 75, 198-203.

[22] Sachithanandan, A, Nanjaiah, P, Nightingale, P, et al. Deep sternal wound infection
requiring revision surgery: impact on mid-term survival following cardiac surgery.
Eur J Cardiothorac Surg (2008). , 33, 673-8.

[23] Pritisanac, A, Gulbins, H, Rosendahl, U, & Ennker, J. Outcome of heart surgery procedures in octogenarians: is age really not an issue? Expert Rev Cardiovasc Ther
(2007).

[24] Prabhakar, G, Haan, C. K, Peterson, E. D, Coombs, L. P, Cruzzavala, J. L, & Murray,
C. F. The risks of moderate and extreme obesity for coronary artery bypass grafting
outcomes: A study from the Society of Thoracic Surgeons' database. Ann Thorac
Surg (2002). , 74, 1125-31.

[25] Furnary, A. P, Zerr, K. J, Grunkemeier, G. L, & Starr, A. Continuous intravenous insulin infusion reduces the incidence of deep sternal wound infection in diabetic patients after cardiac surgical procedures. Ann Thorac Surg (1999). , 67, 352-60.

[26] Halkos, M. E, Puskas, J. D, Lattouf, O. M, et al. Elevated preoperative hemoglobin
A1c level is predictive of adverse events after coronary artery bypass surgery. J Thorac Cardiovasc Surg (2008). , 136, 631-40.

[27] Toumpoulis, I. K, Theakos, N, & Dunning, J. Does bilateral internal thoracic artery
harvest increase the risk of mediastinitis? Interact Cardiovasc Thorac Surg (2007). , 6,
787-91.

[28] De Paulis, R, De Notaris, S, Scaffa, R, et al. The effect of bilateral internal thoracic artery harvesting on superficial and deep sternal infection: the role of skeletonization. J
Thorac Cardiovasc Surg (2005). , 129, 536-43.

[29] Curtis, J. J, Clark, N. C, Mckenney, C. A, et al. Tracheostomy: a risk factor for mediastinitis after cardiac operation. Annals of Thoracic Surgery (2001). , 72, 731-734.

[30] Rahmanian, P. B, Adams, D. H, Castillo, J. G, et al. Tracheostomy is not a risk factor for deep sternal wound infection after cardiac surgery. Annals of Thoracic Surgery (2007). , 84, 1984-1991.

[31] Hubncr, N, Rees, W, Seufert, K, et al. Percutaneous dilatational tracheostomy done early after cardiac surgery-outcome and incidence of mediastinitis. The Thoracic and Cardiovascular Surgeon (1998). , 46, 89-92.

[32] Diehl, J. L, El Atrous, S, Touchard, D, et al. Changes in the work of breathing induced by tracheotomy in ventilator-dependent patients. American Journal of Respiratory and Critical Care Medicine (1999). , 159, 383-388.

[33] Banbury, M. K, Brizzio, M. E, Rajeswaran, J, et al. Transfusion increases the risk of postoperative infection after cardiovascular surgery. Journal of the American College of Surgeons (2006). , 202, 131-138.

[34] Gardlund, B, Bitkover, C, & Vaage, J. Postoperative mediastinitis in cardiac surgery microbiology and pathogenesis. Eur J Cardiothorac Surg (2002). , 21, 825-30.

[35] Mekontso-dessap, A, Kirsch, M, Brun-buisson, C, & Loisance, D. Poststernotomy mediastinitis due to Staphylococcus aureus: comparison of methicillin-resistant and methicillin-susceptible cases. Clin Infect Dis (2001). , 32, 877-83.

[36] San Juan R, Chaves F, López Gude MJ, Díaz-Pedroche C, Otero J, Cortina Romero JM, Rufilanchas JJ, Aguado JM.Staphylococcus aureus poststernotomy mediastinitis: description of two distinct acquisition pathways with different potential preventive approaches. J Thorac Cardiovasc Surg. (2007). , 134, 670-6.

[37] Jakob, H. G, Borneff-lipp, M, Bach, A, et al. The endogenous pathway is a major route for deep sternal wound infection. European Journal of Cardio-Thoracic Surgery (2000). , 17, 154-160.

[38] Kluytmans, J. A, Mouton, J. W, Ijzerman, E. P, et al. Nasal carriage of Staphylococcus aureus as a major risk factor for wound infections after cardiac surgery. The Journal of Infectious Diseases (1995). , 171, 216-219.

[39] Von Eiff, C, Becker, K, Machka, K, Stammer, H, & Peters, G. Nasal carriage as a source of Staphylococcus aureus bacteremia. Study Group. N Engl J Med (2001). , 344, 11-16.

[40] San Juan R, Aguado JM, López MJ, et al. Accuracy of blood culture for early diagnosis of mediastinitis in febrile patients after cardiac surgery. Eur J Clin Microbiol Infect Dis. (2005). , 2005, 24-182.

[41] Tegnell, A, Aren, C, & Ohman, L. Coagulase-negative staphylococi and sternal infections after cardiac operation. Ann Thorac Surg (2000). , 69, 1104-9.

[42] Mekontso Dessap A, Vivier E, Girou E, Brun-Buisson C, Kirsch M.Effect of time to onset on clinical features and prognosis of post-sternotomy mediastinitis. Clin Microbiol Infect (2011). , 17, 292-9.

[43] Jonkers, D, Elenbaas, T, Terporten, P, et al. Prevalence of 90 days postoperative wound infections after cardiac surgery. European Journal of Cardio-Thoracic Surgery (2003). , 23, 97-102.

[44] Mekontso-dessap, A, Kirsch, M, Brun-buisson, C, & Loisance, D. Poststernotomy mediastinitis due to Staphylococcus aureus: comparison of methicillin-resistant and methicillin-susceptible cases. Clin Infect Dis. (2001). , 32, 877-83.

[45] Mauermann, W. J, & Sampathkumar, P. Sternal wound infection. Best Practice & Research Clinical Anaesthesiology (2008). , 22, 423-436.

[46] Baillot, R, Cloutier, D, Montalin, L, et al. Impact of deep sternal wound infection management with vacuum-assisted closure therapy followed by sternal osteosynthesis: a 15-year review of 23,499 sternotomies. Eur J Cardiothorac Surg (2010). , 37, 880-7.

[47] Speir, A. M, Kasirajan, V, Barnett, S. D, & Fonner, E. Jr. Additive costs of postoperative complications for isolated coronary artery bypass grafting patients in Virginia. Ann Thorac Surg (2009). , 88, 40-6.

[48] De Feo, M, Renzulli, A, Ismeno, G, & Gregorio, R. Della Corte A, Utili R, et al. Variables predicting adverse outcome in patients with deep sternal wound infection. *Ann Thorac Surg* (2001). , 71, 324-331.

[49] Graf, K, Ott, E, Vonberg, R. P, Kuehn, C, Haverich, A, & Chaberny, I. F. Economic aspects of deep sternal wound infections. Eur J Cardiothorac Surg (2010). , 37, 893-6.

[50] Ennker, I. C, Kojcici, B, Ennker, J, Vogt, P, & Melichercik, J. Examination of the opportunity costs and turnover situation in patients with deep sternal infections. Zentralbl Chir (2012). , 137, 257-61.

[51] Moidl, R, Fleck, T, Giovanoli, P, Grabenwöger, M, & Wolner, E. Cost effectiveness of V.A.C. therapy after post-sternotomy mediastinitis. Zentralbl Chir (2006). S, 189-90.

[52] Mokhtari, A, Sjögren, J, Nilsson, J, Gustafsson, R, Malmsjö, M, & Ingemansson, R. The cost of vacuum-assisted closure therapy in treatment of deep sternal wound infection. Scand Cardiovasc J (2008). , 42, 85-89.

[53] Atkins, Z. B, & Wolfe, G. Sternal Wound Complications Following Cardiac Surgery. In: Cuneyt N. (ed). Special topics in cardiac surgery. Rijeka, InTech; , 284-308.

[54] Lazar, H. L, Chipkin, S. R, Fitzgerald, C. A, Bao, Y, Cabral, H, & Apstein, C. S. Tight glycemiccontrol in diabetic coronary artery bypass graft patients improves perioperativeoutcomes and decreases recurrent ischemic events. Circulation (2004). , 109, 1497-502.

[55] Gandhi, G. Y, Nuttall, G. A, Abel, M. D, Mullany, C. J, Schaff, H. V, Brien, O, Johnson, P. C, Williams, M. G, Cutshall, A. R, Mundy, S. M, Rizza, L. M, & Mcmahon, R. A. MM. Intensive intraoperative insulin therapy versus conventional glucose management during cardiac surgery: a randomized trial. Ann Intern Med. 200;, 146, 233-43.

[56] Bratzler, D. W, Houck, P. M, Richards, C, Steele, L, et al. Use of antimicrobial prophylaxis for major surgery: baseline results from the National Surgical Infection Prevention Project. Arch Surg. (2005). , 140, 174-82.

[57] Finkelstein, R, Rabino, G, Mashiah, T, et al. Vancomycin versus cefazolin prophylaxis for cardiac surgery in the setting of a high prevalence of methicillin-resistant staphylococcal infections. The Journal of Thoracicand Cardiovascular Surgery (2002). , 123, 326-332.

[58] Bolon, M. K, Morlote, M, Weber, S. G, et al. Glycopeptides are no more effective than beta-lactam agents for prevention of surgical site infection after cardiac surgery: a meta-analysis. Clinical Infectious Diseases (2004). , 38, 1357-1363.

[59] Friberg, O, Svedjeholm, R, Soderquist, B, Granfeldt, H, Vikerfors, T, & Kallman, J. Local gentamicin reduces sternal wound infections after cardiac surgery: a randomized controlled trial. Ann Thorac Surg (2005). , 79, 153-61.

[60] Friberg, O, Dahlin, L. G, Källman, J, Kihlström, E, Söderquist, B, & Svedjeholm, R. Collagen-gentamicin implant for prevention of sternal wound infection; long-term follow-up of effectiveness.Interact Cardiovasc Thorac Surg. (2009). , 9, 454-8.

[61] Bennett-guerrero, E. Ferguson TB Jr, Lin M, Garg J, Mark DB, Scavo VA Jr et al. SWIPE-1 Trial Group. Effect of an implantable gentamicin-collagen sponge on sternal wound infections following cardiac surgery: a randomized trial. J Am Med Assoc (2010). , 304, 755-62.

[62] Mavros, M. N, Mitsikostas, P. K, Alexiou, V. G, Peppas, G, & Falagas, M. E. Gentamicin collagen sponges for the prevention of sternal wound infection: A meta-analysis of randomized controlled trials. J Thorac Cardiovasc Surg. (2012). , 144, 1235-40.

[63] Kaiser, A. B, Kernodle, D. S, Barg, N. L, et al. Influence of preoperative showers on staphylococcal skin colonization: a comparative trial of antiseptic skin cleansers. Annals of Thoracic Surgery (1988). , 45, 35-38.

[64] Byrne DNA, Cuschieri A. The value of whole body disinfection in the prevention of post-operative wound infection in clean and potentially contaminated surgery. Surgical Research Communications (1992). , 12, 43-52.

[65] Perl, T. M, & Golub, J. E. New approaches to reduce Staphylococcus aureus nosocomial infection rates:treating S. aureus nasal carriage. Annals of Pharmacotherapy (1998). S, 7-16.

[66] Cimochowski, G. E, Harostock, M. D, Brown, R, et al. Intranasal mupirocin reduces sternal wound infection after open heart surgery in diabetics and nondiabetics. Annals of Thoracic Surgery (2001). , 71, 1572-1578.

[67] Konvalinka, A, Errett, L, & Fong, I. W. Impact of treating Staphylococcus aureus nasal carriers on wound infections in cardiac surgery. J Hosp Infect. (2006). , 64, 162-8.

[68] Graf, K, Sohr, D, Haverich, A, Kühn, C, Gastmeier, P, & Chaberny, I. F. Decrease of deep sternal surgical site infection rates after cardiac surgery by a comprehensive infection control program. Interact Cardiovasc Thorac Surg. (2009). , 9, 282-6.

[69] Saso, S, James, D, Vecht, J. A, Kidher, E, Kokotsakis, J, Malinovski, V, Rao, C, Darzi, A, Anderson, J. R, & Athanasiou, T. Effect of skeletonization of the internal thoracic artery for coronary revascularization on the incidence of sternal wound infection. Ann Thorac Surg (2010). , 89, 661-70.

[70] Hirose, H, Amano, A, Takanashi, S, & Takahashi, A. Skeletonized bilateral internal mammary artery grafting for patients with diabetes. Interact Cardiovasc Thorac Surg (2003). , 2, 287-92.

[71] Baskett RJF, MacDougall CE, Ross DB. Is mediastinitis a preventable complication? A 10-year review. Ann Thorac Surg (1999). , 67, 462-5.

[72] Robicsek, F, Daugherty, H. K, & Cook, J. W. The prevention and treatment of sternum separartion following open-heart surgery J Thorac Cardiovasc Surg (1977). , 73, 267-268.

[73] Sharma, R, Puri, D, Panigrahi, B. P, & Virdi, I. S. A modified parasternal wire technique for prevention and treatment of sternal dehiscence Ann Thorac Surg (2004). , 77, 210-213.

[74] Friberg, Ö, Dahlin, L. G, Söderquist, B, Källman, J, & Svedjeholm, R. Influence of more than six sternal fixation wires on the incidence of deep sternal wound infection Thorac Cardiovasc Surg (2006). , 54, 468-473.

[75] Schimmer, C, Reents, W, Berneder, S, et al. Prevention of sternal dehiscence and infection in high-risk patients: a prospective randomized multicenter trial. Ann Thorac Surg (2008). , 86, 1897-904.

[76] Plass, A, Emmert, M. Y, Pilsl, M, Salzberg, S. P, Genoni, M, Falk, V, & Grunenfelder, J. Sternal plate closure: indications, surgical procedure and follow-up. Thorac Cardiovasc Surg (2011). , 59, 30-3.

[77] Raman, J, Lehmann, S, Zehr, K, et al. Sternal Closure With Rigid Plate Fixation Versus Wire Closure: A Randomized Controlled Multicenter Trial. Ann Thorac Surg. (2012). doi:pii:S0003-4975(12)01863-2. 0.1016/j.athoracsur.2012.07.085. [Epub ahead of print]

[78] Negri, A, Manfredi, J, Terrini, A, Rodella, G, Bisleri, G, El Quarra, S, & Muneretto, C. Prospective evaluation of a new sternal closure method with thermoreactive clips. Eur J Cardiothorac Surg (2002). , 22, 571-5.

[79] Snyder, C. W, Graham, L. A, Byers, R. E, & Holman, W. L. Primary sternal plating to prevent sternal wound complications after cardiac surgery: early experience and patterns of failure. Interact CardioVasc Thorac Surg (2009). , 9, 763-766.

[80] Bennett-guerrero, E, Phillips-bute, B, Waweru, P. M, Gaca, J. G, Spann, J. C, & Milano, C. A. Pilot study of sternal plating for primary closure of the sternum in cardiac surgical patients. Innovations. (2011). , 6, 382-8.

[81] http://www.kci1.com/KCI1/prevena

[82] Stannard, J. P, Atkins, B. Z, Malley, O, Singh, D, Bernstein, H, Fahey, B, Masden, M, & Attinger, D. CE. Use of negative pressure therapy on closed surgical incisions: a case series. Ostomy Wound Management (2009). , 55, 58-66.

[83] Wackenfors, A, Sjögren, J, Gustafsson, R, Algotsson, L, Ingemansson, R, & Malmsjö, M. Effects of vacuum-assisted closure therapy on inguinal wound edge microvascular blood flow. Wound Repair Regen (2004). , 12, 600-6.

[84] Colli, A. First experience with a new negative pressure incision management system on surgical incisions after cardiac surgery in high risk patients. Journal of Cardiothoracic Surgery (2011).

[85] Atkins, B. Z, Wooten, M. K, Kistler, J, Hurley, K, & Hughes, G. C. Wolfe WG: Does negative pressure wound therapy have a role in preventing poststernotomy wound complications? Surg Innov (2009).

[86] Robicsek, F. Postoperative Sterno-mediastinitis. Am Surg (2000). , 66, 184-192.

[87] Sarr, M. G, Gott, V. L, & Townsend, T. R. Mediastinal infection after cardiac surgery. Ann Thorac Surg (1984).

[88] Shumacker, H. B, & Mandelbaum, I. Continuous antibiotic irrigation in the treatment of infection. Arch Surg (1963).

[89] Merrill, W. H, Akhter, S. A, Wolf, R. K, & Schneeberger, E. W. Flege JB Jr. Simplified treatment of postoperative mediastinitis..Ann Thorac Surg. (2004). , 78, 608-12.

[90] .Poncelet, A. J, Lengele, B, Delaere, B, et al. Algorithm for primary closure in sternal wound infection: a single institution 10-year experience. Eur J Cardiothorac Surg. (2008). , 33, 232-8.

[91] Kirsch, M, Mekontso-dessap, A, Houël, R, Giroud, E, Hillion, M. L, & Loisance, D. Y. Closed drainage using redon catheters for poststernotomy mediastinitis: results and risk factors for adverse outcome.. Ann Thorac Surg. (2001). , 71, 1580-6.

[92] Levi, N, & Olsen, P. S. Primary closure of deep sternal wound infection following open heart surgery: a safe operation? J Cardiovasc Surg (Torino). (2000). Apr;, 41(2), 241-5.

[93] Lee, A. B, Schimert, G, Shaktin, S, et al. Total excision of the sternum and thoracic pedicle transposition of the greater omentum; useful stratagems in managing severe mediastinal infection following open heart surgery. Surgery (1976). , 80, 433-6.

[94] Jurkiewicz, M. J, Bostwick, J, Hester, T. R, et al. Infected median sternotomy wound: successful treatment by muscle flaps. Ann Surg (1980).

[95] Jones, G, Jurkiewicz, M. J, et al. Management of the infected median sternotomy wound with muscle flaps. Ann Surg (1997). , 225, 766-78.

[96] Brandt, C, & Alvarez, J. M. First-line treatment of deep sternal infection by a plastic surgical approach: superior results compared with conventional cardiac surgical orthodoxy. Plast Reconstr Surg. (2002). , 109, 2231-7.

[97] Wong CHK, Senewiratne S, Garlick G, Mullany D. Two-stage management of sternal wound infection using bilateral pectoralis major advancement flap. Eur J Cardiothorac Surg (2006). , 30, 148-152.

[98] Milano, C. A, Georgiade, G, Muhlbaier, L. H, Smith, P. K, & Wolfe, W. G. Comparison of omental and pectoralis flaps for poststernotomy mediastinitis. Ann Thorac Surg (1999). , 67, 377-81.

[99] El Oakley, R. M, & Wright, J. E. Postoperative mediastinitis: classification and management. Ann Thorac Surg (1996). , 61, 1030-6.

[100] Molina, E. Primary closure for infected dehiscence of the sternum. Ann Thorac Surg (1993). , 55, 459-63.

[101] Scully, H. E, Leclerc, Y, Martin, R. D, et al. Comparison between antibiotic irrigation and mobilization of pectoral muscle flaps in treatment of deep sternal infection. J Thorac Cardiovasc Surg (1985). , 90, 523-31.

[102] Rand, R. P, Cochran, R. P, Aziz, S, Hofer, B. O, Allen, M. D, Verrier, E. D, et al. Prospective trial of catheter irrigation and muscle flaps for sternal wound infection. *Ann Thorac Surg* (1998). , 65, 1046-1049.

[103] Ringelman, P. R, Vander, K. C, Cameron, D, Bumgartner, W. A, & Manson, P. N. Long-term results of flap reconstruction in median sternotomy wound infection. Plast Reconstr Surg (1994). , 93, 1208-14.

[104] Pairolero, P. C, & Arnold, P. C. Management of recalcitrant median sternotomy wounds. J Thorac Cardiovasc Surg (1984). , 88, 357-64.

[105] Levi, N, & Olsen, P. S. Primary closure of deep sternal wound infection following open heart surgery: a safe operation? J Cardiovasc Surg (Torino). (2000). , 41, 241-5.

[106] Nahai, F, Rand, R. P, Hester, T. R, et al. Primary treatment of the infected sternotomy wound with muscle flaps: a review of 211 consecutive cases. Plast Reconstr Surg (1989)., 84, 434-441.

[107] Kutsal, A, Ibrisim, E, Catav, Z, et al. Mediastinitis after open heart surgery. Analysis of risk factors and management. J Cardiovasc Surg (Torino) (1991)., 32, 38-41.

[108] Van Wingerden, J. J, Coret, M. E, Van Nieuwenhoven, C. A, & Totté, E. R. The laparoscopically harvested omental flap for deep sternal wound infection. Eur J Cardiothorac Surg (2010)., 37, 87-92.

[109] Atkins, B. Z, Onaitis, M. W, Hutcheson, K. A, Kaye, K, Petersen, R. P, & Wolfe, W. G. Does method of sternal repair influence long-term outcome of postoperative mediastinitis? Am J Surg. (2011)., 202, 565-7.

[110] Christian, M. The role of hyperbaric oxygen therapy in the treatment of sternal wound infectionEur J Cardiothorac Surg (2006)., 30, 153-159.

[111] Siondalski, P, Keita, L, Sicko, Z, Zelechowski, P, Jaworski, L, & Rogowski, J. Surgical treatment and adjunct hyperbaric therapy to improve healing of wound infection complications after sterno-mediastinitis. Pneumonol Alergol Pol (2003)., 71, 12-16.

[112] Obdeijn, M. C, De Lange, M. Y, Lichtendahl, D. H, & De Boer, W. J. Vacuum-assisted closure in the treatment of poststernotomy mediastinitis. Ann Thorac Surg (1999)., 68, 2358-60.

[113] Catarino, P. A, Chamberlain, M. H, Wright, N. C, Black, E, Campbell, K, Robson, D, & Pillai, R. G. High-pressure suction drainage via a polyurethane foam in the management of poststernotomy mediastinitis. Ann Thorac Surg (2000)., 70, 1891-5.

[114] Gustafsson, R. I, Sjögren, J, & Ingemansson, R. Deep sternal wound infection: a sternal-sparing technique with vacuum-assisted closure therapy. Ann Thorac Surg. (2003)., 76, 2048-53.

[115] Fleck, T. M, Fleck, M, Moidl, R, et al. The vacuum-assisted closure system for the treatment of deep sternal wound infections after cardiac surgery. Ann Thorac Surg (2002)., 74, 1596-600.

[116] Sjögren, J, Gustafsson, R, Nilsson, J, Lindstedt, S, Nozohoor, S, & Ingemansson, R. Negative-pressure wound therapy following cardiac surgery: bleeding complications and 30-day mortality in 176 patients with deep sternal wound infection. Interact Cardiovasc Thorac Surg (2011)., 12, 117-20.

[117] Fleck, T, Moidl, R, Giovanoli, P, et al. A conclusion from the first 125 patients treated with the vacuum assisted closure system for postoperative sternal wound infection. Interact Cardiovasc Thorac Surg. (2006)., 5, 145-8.

[118] Ennker, I. C, Malkoc, A, Pietrowski, D, Vogt, P. M, Ennker, J, & Albert, A. The concept of negative pressure wound therapy (NPWT) after poststernotomy mediastinitis--a single center experience with 54 patients. J Cardiothorac Surg. (2009). Jan 12;4:5.

[119] Šimek, M, Kaláb, M, Molitor, M, et al. Topical negative pressure in the treatment of deep sternal infection following cardiac surgery: 5-year results of first-line application protocol. The EWMA Journal (2011). , 11, 38-41.

[120] Gustafsson, R, Johnsson, P, Algotsson, L, Blomquist, S, & Ingemansson, R. Vacuum-assisted closure therapy guided by C-reactive protein level in patients with deep sternal wound infection. J Thorac Cardiovasc Surg (2002). , 123, 895-900.

[121] Berg, H. F. Brands WGB, Geldrop van TR, Kluytmans-VandenBergh MFQ, Kluytmans JAJW. Comparison between closed drainage techniques for the treatment of postoperative mediastinitis. Ann Thorac Surg (2000). , 70, 924-929.

[122] Doss, M, Martens, S, Wood, J. P, Wolff, J. D, & Baier, C. Moritz. Vacuum-assisted suction drainage versus conventional treatment in the management of poststernotomy osteomyelitis Eur J Cardiothorac Surg (2002). , 22, 934-938.

[123] Song, D. H, Wu, L. C, Lohman, R. F, Gottlieb, L. J, & Franczyk, M. Vacuum-assisted closure for the treatment of sternal wounds: the bridge between debridement and definitive closure. Plast Reconstr Surg (2003). , 111, 92-97.

[124] Luckraz, H, Murphy, F, Bryant, S, Charman, S, & Ritchie, A. Vacuum-assisted closure as a treatment modality for infections after cardiac surgery J Thorac Cardiovasc Surg (2003). , 125, 301-305.

[125] Fuchs, U, Zittermann, A, Stuetten, B, Groening, A, Minami, K, & Koefer, R. Clinical outcome of patients with deep sternal infection managed by vacuum-assisted closure compared to conventional therapy with open packing: A retrospective analysis. Ann Thorac Surg (2005). , 79, 526-31.

[126] Sjögren, J, Gustafsson, R, Nilsson, J, Malmsjö, M, & Ingemansson, R. Clinical outcome after poststernotomy mediastinitis: vacuum-assisted closure versus conventional treatment. Ann Thorac Surg. (2005). , 79, 2049-55.

[127] Immer, F. F, Durrer, M, Mühlemann, K. S, Erni, D, Gahl, B, & Carrel, T. P. Deep sternal wound infection after cardiac surgery: modality of treatment and outcome. Ann Thorac Surg. (2005). , 80, 957-61.

[128] Segers, P, De Jong, A. P, & Kloek, J. J. de Mol BAJM. Poststernotomy mediastinitis: comparison of two treatment modalities. Interact Cardiovasc Thorac Surg (2005). , 4, 555-560.

[129] Petzina, R, Hoffmann, J, Navasardyan, A, et al. Negative pressure wound therapy for post-sternotomy mediastinitis reduces mortality rate and sternal re-infection rate compared to conventional treatment.Eur J Cardiothorac Surg (2010). , 38, 110-3.

[130] Simek, M, Hajek, R, Fluger, I, et al. Superiority of topical negative pressure over closed irrigation therapy of deep sternal wound infection in cardiac surgery. J Cardiovasc Surg (Torino) (2012). , 53, 113-20.

[131] De Feo, M. Della Corte A, Vicchio M, Pirozzi F, Nappi G, Cotrufo M. Is post-sternotomy mediastinitis still devastating after the advent of negative-pressure wound therapy? Tex Heart Inst J (2011). , 38, 375-80.

[132] Assmann, A, Boeken, U, Feindt, P, Schurr, P, Akhyari, P, & Lichtenberg, A. Vacuum-assisted wound closure is superior to primary rewiring in patients with deep sternal woundinfection. Thorac Cardiovasc Surg (2011). , 59, 25-9.

[133] Vos, R. J, Yilmaz, A, Sonker, U, Kelder, J. C, & Kloppenburg, G. T. Vacuum-assisted closure of post-sternotomy mediastinitis as compared to open packing. Interact Cardiovasc Thorac Surg. (2012). , 14, 17-21.

[134] Deniz, H, Gokaslan, G, Arslanoglu, Y, Ozcaliskan, O, Guzel, G, Yasim, A, & Ustunsoy, H. Treatment outcomes of postoperative mediastinitis in cardiac surgery; negative pressure wound therapy versus conventional treatment. J Cardiothorac Surg (2012).

[135] Fleck, T, & Fleck, M. Negative pressure wound therapy for the treatment of sternal wound infections after cardiac surgery. Int Wound J (2012). doi:j.X.2012.01079.x. [Epub ahead of print], 1742-481.

[136] Raja, S. G, & Berg, G. A. Should vacuum-assisted closure therapy be routinely used for management of deep sternal wound infection after cardiac surgery?Interact CardioVasc Thorac Surg (2007). , 6-523.

[137] Schimmer, C, Sommer, S. P, Bensch, M, Elert, O, & Leyh, R. Management of poststernotomy mediastinitis: experience and results of different therapy modalities.Thorac Cardiovasc Surg. (2008). , 56, 200-4.

[138] Damiani, G, Pinnarelli, L, Sommella, L, Tocco, M. P, Marvulli, M, Magrini, P, & Ricciardi, W. Vacuum-assisted closure therapy for patients with infected sternal wounds: a meta-analysis of current evidence. J Plast Reconstr Aesthet Surg (2011). , 64, 1119-23.

[139] De Feo, M, Vicchio, M, Nappi, G, & Cotrufo, M. Role of vacuum in methicillin-resistant deep sternal wound infection.Asian Cardiovasc Thorac Ann. (2010). , 18, 360-3.

[140] Al-ebrahim, K. E. Sternocutaneous fistulas after cardiac surgery. Ann Thorac Surg (2010). , 89, 1705-6.

[141] Gaudreau, G, Costache, V, Houde, C, Cloutier, D, Montalin, L, Voisine, P, & Baillot, R. Recurrent sternal infection following treatment with negative pressure wound therapy and titanium transverse plate fixation. Eur J Cardiothorac Surg. (2010). , 37, 888-92.

[142] Steingrímsson, S, Gustafsson, R, Gudbjartsson, T, Mokhtari, A, Ingemansson, R, & Sjögren, J. Sternocutaneous fistulas after cardiac surgery: incidence and late outcome during a ten-year follow-up. Ann Thorac Surg (2009). , 88, 1910-5.

[143] Darouiche, R. O. Treatment of infections associated with surgical implants.N Engl J Med (2004). , 350, 1422-9.

[144] Bu-omar, Y, Naik, M. J, Catarino, P. A, & Ratnatunga, C. Right ventricular rupture during use of high-pressure suction drainage in the management of poststernotomy mediastinitis. Ann Thorac Surg. (2003).

[145] Bapat, V, Muttardi, N, Young, C, Venn, G, & Roxburgh, J. Experience with Vacuum-assisted closure of sternal wound infections following cardiac surgery and evaluation of chronic complications associated with its use. J Card Surg. (2008). , 23, 227-33.

[146] Van Wingerden, J. J, Segers, P, & Jekel, L. Major bleeding during negative pressure wound/V.A.C.®--therapy for postsurgical deep sternal wound infection--a critical appraisal. J Cardiothorac Surg. 201;6:121.

[147] Hayward, R. H, Korompai, F. L, & Knight, W. L. The open sternotomy wound and risk of acute hemorrhage. J Thorac Cardiovasc Surg (1992). , 103, 1228-30.

[148] Khoynezhad, A, Abbas, G, Palazzo, R. S, & Graver, L. M. Spontaneous right ventricular disruption following treatment of sternal infection. J Card Surg (2004). , 19, 74-8.

[149] Niclauss, L, Delay, D, & Stumpe, F. Right ventricular rupture due to recurrent mediastinal infection with a closed chest. Interact Cardiovasc Thorac Surg (2010). , 10, 470-2.

[150] Petzina, R, Malmsjö, M, Stamm, C, & Hetzer, R. Major complications during negative pressure wound therapy in poststernotomy mediastinitis after cardiac surgery. J Thorac Cardiovasc Surg.(2010). , 140, 1133-6.

[151] Malmsjö, M, Petzina, R, Ugander, M, Engblom, H, Torbrand, C, Mokhtari, A, Hetzer, R, Arheden, H, & Ingemansson, R. Preventing heart injury during negative pressure wound therapy in cardiac surgery: assessment using real-time magnetic resonance imaging. J Thorac Cardiovasc Surg (2009). , 138, 712-7.

[152] Voss, B, Bauernschmitt, R, Will, A, et al. Sternal reconstruction with titanium plates in complicated sternal dehiscence. Eur J Cardiothorac Surg (2008). , 34, 139-145.

[153] Gaudreau, G, Costache, V, Houde, C, Cloutier, D, Montalin, L, Voisine, P, & Baillot, R. Recurrent sternal infection following treatment with negative pressure wound therapy and titanium transverse plate fixation. Eur J Cardiothorac Surg (2010). , 37, 888-92.

[154] Voss, B, Bauernschmitt, R, Brockmann, G, et al. Osteosynthetic thoracic stabilization after complete resection of sternum. Eur J Cardiothorac Surg (2007). , 32, 391-393.

[155] Piotrowski, J. A, Fischer, M, Klaes, W, & Splittgerber, F. Autologous bone transplant after sternal resection. J Cardiovasc Surg (Torino) (1996). , 37, 179-81.

[156] Nahabedian, M. Y, Riley, L. H, Greene, P. S, et al. Sternal stabilization using allograft fibula following cardiac transplantation. Plastic Reconstr Surg (2001). , 108, 1284-8.

[157] Marulli, G, Hamad, A. M, Cogliati, E, Breda, C, Zuin, A, & Rea, F. Allograft sterno-chondral replacement after resection of large sternal chondrosarcoma. J Thorac Cardiovasc Surg (2010). e, 69-70.

[158] Dell'amore A, Cassanelli N, Dolci G, Stella F.An alternative technique for anterior chest wall reconstruction: the sternal allograft transplantation. Interact Cardiovasc ThoracInteract Cardiovasc Thorac Surg. (2012). , 15, 944-7.

[159] Dell'Amore A, Dolci G, Cassanelli N, Bini A, Stella F.A massive post-sternotomy sternal defect treated by allograft sternal transplantation. J Card Surg (2012). , 27, 557-9.

[160] Kalab, M, Molitor, M, Kubesova, B, & Lonsky, V. Use of allogenous bone graft and osteosynthetic stabilization in treatment of massive post-sternotomy defects. Eur J Cardiothorac Surg. (2012). Jun;41(6):e, 182-4.

[161] Collection of Laws of The Czech RepublicAct (2008). Collegium on Human Tissues and Cells. Prague, 2008.(296)

[162] European Association of Tissue BanksGeneral Standards for Tissue Banking. ÖBIG-Transplant, Vienna, (1995).

[163] Perkins, D. J, Hunt, J. A, Pennington, D. G, & Stern, H. S. Secondary sternal repair following median sternotomy using interosseous absorbable sutures and pectoralis major myocutaneous advancement flaps. British J Plast Surg (1996). , 49, 214-219.

[164] Brito, J. D, Assumpcao, C. R, Murad, H, & Jazbik, A. P. Sa MPL, Bastos ES, Giambroni Filho R, Silva RS. One-stage management of infected sternotomy wounds using bilateral pectoralis major myocutaneous advancement flap. Rev Bras Cir Cardiovasc (2009). , 24, 58-63.

[165] Greig AVH, Geh JLC, Khanduja V, Shibu M.Choice of flap for the management of deep sternal wound infection- an anatomical classification. J Plast Reconstr Aesth Surg. (2007). , 60, 372-378.

[166] Salgado, C. J, Mardini, S, Mamali, A. A, Ortiz, J, Gonzales, R, & Chen, H. C. Muscle versus nonmuscle flaps in the reconstructon of chronic osteomyelitis defects. Plast Reconstr Surg, (2006). , 118, 1401-1411.

[167] Yazar, S, Lin, Y. T, Ulusal, A. E, & Wei, F. C. Outcome comparison between free muscle and free fasciocutaneous flaps for reconstruction of distal third and ankle traumatic opetn tibial fractures. Plast Reconstr Surg, (2006). , 117, 2468-2475.

[168] Serafin, D. The Pectoralis Major Muscle Flap. In Serafin D. Atlas of Microsurgical Composite Tissue Tranplantation. W.B.Saunders company, London, (1996). , 1996, 161-174.

[169] Netscher, D. T, Eladoumikdachi, F, Mchugh, P. M, Thornby, J, & Soltero, E. Sternal wound debridement and muscle flap reconstruction: functional implications. Annals of Plast Surg (2003). , 51, 115-122.

[170] Cohen, M, Yaniv, Y, Weiss, J, Greif, J, Gur, E, Wertheym, E, & Shafir, R. Median sternotomy wound complication: the effect of reconstruction on lung function. Annals Plast Surg (1997). , 39, 36-43.

[171] Arnold, P. G, & Pairolero, P. C. Chest-wall reconstruction. An account of 500 consecutive patients. Plast Reconstr Surg (1996). , 98, 804-810.

[172] Skoracki, R. J, & Chang, D. W. Reconstruction of the chestwall and thorax. J Surg Oncol (2006). , 94, 455-465.

[173] Ascherman, J. A, Patel, S. M, Malhotra, S. M, & Smith, C. R. Management of sternla wounds with bilateral pectoralis major myocutaneous advancement flaps in 114 consecutively treated patients: refinements in technique and outcomes analysis. Plast Reconstr Surg (2004). , 114, 676-83.

[174] Hugo, N. E, Sultan, M. R, Ascherman, J. A, Patsis, M. C, Smith, C. R, & Rose, E. A. Single-stage management of 74 consecutive sternla wound complications with pectoralis major myocutaneous advancement flaps. Plast Reconstr Surg (1994). , 93, 1433-1441.

[175] Brutus, J. P, Nikolis, A, Perreault, I, & Harris, P. G. The unilateralpectoralis major island flap, an efficient and straightforward procedure for reconstruction of full length sternal defects after postoperative mediastinal wound infection. Brit J Plast Surg (2004). , 57, 803-805.

[176] Chou, E, Tai, Y, Chen, I I, & Chen, K. Simple and reliable way in sternum wound coverage-tripedicle pectoralis major musculocutaneous flap. Microsurgery. (2008). , 28, 441-6.

[177] Majure, J. A, Albin, R. E, Donnell, O, & Arganese, R. S. TJ. Reconstruction of the infected median sternotomy wound. Ann Thorac Surg (1986). , 42, 9-12.

[178] Molitor, M, Simek, M, Lonský, V, Kaláb, M, Veselý, J, & Zálešák, B. Pectoral muscle flap with v-y skin paddle for covering sternal defects. Ann Thorac Surg. (2012). e, 131-3.

[179] Hallock, G. G. The breast musculocutaneous flap for complete coverage of the median sternotomy wound. Plast Reconstr Surg (2003). , 112, 199-203.

[180] Nahai, F, Morales, L, Bone, D. K, & Botswick, J. Pectoralis Major Muscle Turnover Flaps for Closure of the infected Sternotomy Wound with Preservation of Form and Function. Plast Reconstr Surg (1982). , 70, 471-474.

[181] Spiess, A. M, Balakrishnan, C. H, & Gursel, E. Fascial release of the pectoralis major:a technique used in pectoralis major muscle closure of the mediastinum in cases of mediastinitis. Plast Reconstr Surg. (2007). , 119, 573-7.

[182] Serafin, D. The Pectoralis Major Muscle Flap. In Serafin D. Atlas of Microsurgical Composite Tissue Tranplantation. W.B.Saunders company, London, (1996). , 1996, 221-247.

[183] Skoracki, R. J, & Chang, D. W. Reconstruction of the chestwall and thorax. J Surg Oncol. (2006). Review., 94, 455-65.

[184] Acinapura, A. J, Godfrey, N, Romita, M, Cunningham, J, Adams, P. X, Jacobowitz, I. S, Rose, D. M, & Nealon, T. Surgical management of infected median sternotomy:Closed irrigation vs muscle flaps. J Cardiovasc. Surg (1985). , 26, 443-446.

[185] Ford, T. D. Rectus abdominis myocutaneous flap used to close a median sternotomy chest defect. S Afr Med J (1985). , 68, 115-116.

[186] Solomon, M. P, & Granick, M. S. Bipedicle muscle flaps in sternal wound repair. Plast Reconstr Surg. (1998). , 101, 356-6.

[187] Laitung JKG, Peck F. Shoulder function following the loss of the latissimus dorsi muscle. British J Plast Surg (1985). , 38, 375-379.

[188] Dejesus, R. A, Paletta, J. D, & Dabb, R. W. Reconstruction of the median sternotomy sound dehiscence using the latissimus dorsi myocutaneous flap. J Cardiovasc Surg (2001). , 42, 359-564.

[189] Fansa, H, Handstein, S, & Schneider, W. Treatment of infected median sternotomy wounds with a myocutaneous latissimus dorsi muscle flap. Scand Cardiovasc J (1998). , 32, 33-39.

[190] Roshan, A, Kotwal, A, & Riaz, M. Stanley PRW. Sternal wound dehiscence complicated by macromastia: report of two cases with discussion of literature. J Plast Reconstr Aesth Surg (2009). ee364., 362.

[191] Copeland, M, Senkowski, C, Ergin, A, et al. Macromastia as a factor in sternal wound dehiscence following cardiac surgery:management combining chest wall reconstruction and reduction mammaplasty. J Card Surg (1992). , 7, 275-278.

[192] Fontaine, S, Devos, S, & Goldschmidt, D. Reduction mammoplasty combined with pectoralis major muscle flaps for median sternotomy wound closure. Br J Plats Surg (1996). , 49, 220-222.

[193] Uygur, F, Sever, C, Ulkur, E, & Celikoz, B. Reconstruction of large post-sternotomy wound with bilateral V-Y fasciocutaneous advancement flaps. Ann Thorac Surg (2008). , 86, 1012-1015.

[194] Roshan, A, Kotwal, A, & Riaz, M. Stanley PRW. Sternal wound dehiscence complicated by macromastia: report of two cases with discussion of literature. J Plast Reconstr Aesth Surg (2009). ee364., 362.

[195] Würinger, E, Mader, N, Posch, E, & Holle, J. Nerve and vessel supplying ligamentous suspension of the mammary gland. Plast Reconstr Surg (1998). , 101, 1486-1493.

[196] Hamdi, M, & Dancey, A. The septum-based therapeutic mammaplasty technique for management of sternal defects. Plast Reconstr Surg (2010). , 569-573.

[197] Hughes, K. C, Henry, M. J, Turner, J, & Manders, E. K. Design of the cyclops flap for chest-wall reconstruction. Plast Reconstr Surg (1997). , 100, 1146-51.

[198] Aydin, A, Güven, E, Keklik, B, Basaran, K, & Özkan, B. Reconstruction of the Chest Wall Defects with Mammary Dermoglandular Advancement Flaps in Female Complicated Cases. Trakya Univ Tip Fak Derg (2009). , 26, 130-133.

[199] Yasuura, K, Okamoto, H, Morita, S, Ogawa, Y, Sawazaki, M, Seki, A, Masumoto, H, Matsuura, A, Maseki, T, & Torii, S. Results of omental flap transposition for deep sternal wound infection after cardiovascular surgery. Annals of Surg (1998). , 227, 455-459.

[200] Mathisen, D. J, Grillo, H. C, Vlahakes, G. J, et al. The omentum in the management of complicated cardiothoracic probleme. J Thorac Cardiovasc Surg (1988). , 95, 677-684.

[201] Weinzweig, N, & Hetman, R. Transposition of the greater omentum for recalcitrant median sternotomy wound infection. Annals Plast. Surg (1995). , 34, 471-477.

[202] Alday, E. S, & Golsdmith, H. S. Surgical technique for ometal lenghtening based on arterial anatomy. Surg Gynecol Obstet (1972).

[203] Das, S. K. The size of the human omentum and methods of lenghtening it for transposition. Br J Plast Surg (1976). , 29, 170-174.

[204] Weinzweig, N, & Hetman, R. Transposition of the greater omentum for recalcitrant median sternotomy wound infection. Annals Plast. Surg (1995). , 34, 471-477.

[205] Pearl, S. N, & Dibbell, D. G. Reconstruction after median sternotomy infection. Surg Gynecol Obstet (1984). , 159, 47-52.

[206] Colen, L. B, Huntsman, W. T, & Morain, W. D. The integrated approach to suppurative mediastinitis: rewiring the sternum over transposed omentum. Plast Reconstr Surg (1989). , 84, 936-943.

[207] Hakellus, L. Fatal complication after use of the greater omentum for reconstruction of the chest wall. Plast Reconstr Surg (1978).

[208] Acarturk, T. O, Swartz, W. M, Luketich, J, et al. Laparoscopically harvested omental flap for chest wall and intrathoracic reconstruction. Ann Plast Surg (2004). , 53, 210-216.

[209] Barragan, B. A, Hallodorsson, A. O, Wachtel, M. S, & Frezza, E. E. Laparoscopic greater omentum harvesting with split-thickness skin grafting for sternal wound dehiscence. The American Surgeon (2006). , 72, 829-832.

[210] Reichenberger, M. A, Harenberg, P. S, Pelzer, M, Gazyakan, E, Ryssel, G, Hermann, G, & Engel, H. Arteriovenous loops in microsurgical free tissue transfer in reconstruction of central sternal defects. J Thorac Cardiovasc Surg (2010). , 140, 1283-1287.

[211] Engel, H, Pelzer, M, Sauerbier, M, Hermann, G, & Heitmann, C. An innovative treatment concept for free flap reconstruction of komplex central chest wall defects- the cephalic-thoraco-acromial (CTA) loop. Microsurgery (2007). , 27, 481-486.

Permissions

The contributors of this book come from diverse backgrounds, making this book a truly international effort. This book will bring forth new frontiers with its revolutionizing research information and detailed analysis of the nascent developments around the world.

We would like to thank Wilbert S. Aronow, MD, for lending his expertise to make the book truly unique. He has played a crucial role in the development of this book. Without his invaluable contribution this book wouldn't have been possible. He has made vital efforts to compile up to date information on the varied aspects of this subject to make this book a valuable addition to the collection of many professionals and students.

This book was conceptualized with the vision of imparting up-to-date information and advanced data in this field. To ensure the same, a matchless editorial board was set up. Every individual on the board went through rigorous rounds of assessment to prove their worth. After which they invested a large part of their time researching and compiling the most relevant data for our readers. Conferences and sessions were held from time to time between the editorial board and the contributing authors to present the data in the most comprehensible form. The editorial team has worked tirelessly to provide valuable and valid information to help people across the globe.

Every chapter published in this book has been scrutinized by our experts. Their significance has been extensively debated. The topics covered herein carry significant findings which will fuel the growth of the discipline. They may even be implemented as practical applications or may be referred to as a beginning point for another development. Chapters in this book were first published by InTech; hereby published with permission under the Creative Commons Attribution License or equivalent.

The editorial board has been involved in producing this book since its inception. They have spent rigorous hours researching and exploring the diverse topics which have resulted in the successful publishing of this book. They have passed on their knowledge of decades through this book. To expedite this challenging task, the publisher supported the team at every step. A small team of assistant editors was also appointed to further simplify the editing procedure and attain best results for the readers.

Our editorial team has been hand-picked from every corner of the world. Their multi-ethnicity adds dynamic inputs to the discussions which result in innovative outcomes. These outcomes are then further discussed with the researchers and contributors who give their valuable feedback and opinion regarding the same. The feedback is then collaborated with the researches and they are edited in a comprehensive manner to aid the understanding of the subject.

Apart from the editorial board, the designing team has also invested a significant amount of their time in understanding the subject and creating the most relevant covers. They scrutinized every image to scout for the most suitable representation of the subject and create an appropriate cover for the book.

The publishing team has been involved in this book since its early stages. They were actively engaged in every process, be it collecting the data, connecting with the contributors or procuring relevant information. The team has been an ardent support to the editorial, designing and production team. Their endless efforts to recruit the best for this project, has resulted in the accomplishment of this book. They are a veteran in the field of academics and their pool of knowledge is as vast as their experience in printing. Their expertise and guidance has proved useful at every step. Their uncompromising quality standards have made this book an exceptional effort. Their encouragement from time to time has been an inspiration for everyone.

The publisher and the editorial board hope that this book will prove to be a valuable piece of knowledge for researchers, students, practitioners and scholars across the globe.

List of Contributors

Yuki Igarashi
University of Tsukuba, Japan

Takeo Igarashi
The University of Tokyo, Japan

Ryo Haraguchi and Kazuo Nakazawa
National Cerebral and Cardiovascular Center Research Institute, Japan

Michael Tsang and JD Schwalm
Department of Medicine, Division of Cardiology, McMaster University, Hamilton Health Sciences, Population Health Research Institute, Hamilton, Ontario, Canada

Mohammed Balghith
King Saud Bin Abdulaziz University for Heath Sciences, KACC, National Guard, Riyadh, Saudi Arabia

Takao Kato
Cardiovascular Center, The Tazuke Kofukai Medical Research Institute, Kitano Hospital, Osaka, Japan

Aditya M. Sharma
University of Virginia, Charlottesville, VA, USA

Herbert D. Aronow
St. Joseph Mercy Hospital, Ann Arbor MI, USA

Eduardo Keller Saadi
Federal University of Rio Grande do Sul, Porto Alegre, RS, Brazil Federal University of Rio Grande do Sul Hospital, Porto Alegre, RS, Brazil Mãe de Deus Hospital, Porto Alegre, RS, Brazil

Rui Almeida
West Paraná State University, Cascavel, PR, Brazil Mãe de Deus Hospital, Cascavel, PR, Brazil Cardiovascular Surgery Institute of West Paraná, Cascavel, PR, Brazil

Alexandre do Canto Zago
Federal University of Rio Grande do Sul, Porto Alegre, RS, Brazil Federal University of Rio Grande do Sul Hospital, Porto Alegre, RS, Brazil Lutheran University Hospital, Porto Alegre, RS, Brazil

Muhammad A. Chaudhry
Scripps Green Hospital, La Jolla, California, USA

Zainab Omar
King Edward Medical College, Lahore, Pakistan

Faisal Latif
University of Oklahoma Health Sciences Center, Oklahoma City, Oklahoma, USA

Kim Houlind
Dept. of Vascular Surgery, Kolding Hospital, Denmark and Institute of Regional Health
Services Research, University of Southern Denmark, Denmark

Johnny Christensen
Dept. of Radiology, Kolding Hospital, Denmark

Zsuzsanna Cserép
Department of Anesthesiology and Intensive Care, Semmelweis University, Budapest,
Hungary and Uzsoki Street Hospital of the Budapest Municipality, Budapest, Hungary

Andrea Székely
Department of Anesthesiology and Intensive Care, Semmelweis University, Budapest,
Hungary and Uzsoki Street Hospital of the Budapest Municipality, Budapest, Hungary
Intensive Care, Gottsegen György Hungarian Institute of Cardiology, Budapest, Hungary

Bela Merkely
Department of Cardiology, Semmelweis University, Budapest, Hungary

Martin Šimek, Martin Molitor and Vladimír Lonský
Department of Cardiac Surgery, University Hospital Olomouc, Olomouc, Czech Republic

Martin Kaláb
Department of Plastic Surgery, University Hospital Bulovka, Prague, Czech Republic

Patrick Tobbia
Department of Medicine, Cone Health, University of North Carolina, Greensboro, NC,
USA

Printed in the USA
CPSIA information can be obtained
at www.ICGtesting.com
JSHW011419221024
72173JS00004B/588